THE DR ALKALINE AND ANTI-INFLAMMATORY DIET FOR BEGINNERS

A Step-by-Step Guide to Achieving Lifelong Health by Lowering Your Internal Inflammation

Tasha Chathem

CHAPTER 6: TRANSITIONING TO TRANQUILITY 101

Introduction: The Dawn of Healing

In the realm of health and wellness, there exists an eternal quest for the secrets of longevity, vitality, and well-being. We are all searching for ways to thrive, not just survive, in this fast-paced world. The modern age has brought us incredible advancements in science and medicine, but it has also led to an epidemic of chronic diseases and a disconnection from the natural world. In our journey towards healing and rediscovering the essence of natural well-being, we find a guiding light in the revolutionary insights of Dr. Sebi.

Why This Book

In an age of information overload, where countless health books and self-proclaimed gurus flood the market, it's crucial to understand why this book is unique and essential. The answer lies in the transformative wisdom of Dr. Sebi, who dedicated his life to uncovering the secrets of the natural world and how it can heal us. This book delves into his groundbreaking work, his philosophy, and the principles that can empower you to take control of your health and vitality.

Who Was Dr. Sebi?

Dr. Sebi, whose real name was Alfredo Darrington Bowman, was a controversial figure known for his alternative health practices and dietary recommendations. Born on November 26, 1933, in Ilanga, Honduras, Dr.

Sebi gained notoriety for his claims to have discovered a natural, holistic approach to healing various health conditions through nutrition and herbal remedies. His work primarily revolved around the concept that certain foods and substances could cleanse and detoxify the body, leading to improved health & vitality. While Dr. Sebi had a dedicated following and was seen as a visionary by some, he also faced skepticism and criticism from the medical community and regulatory authorities.

Early Life and Background

Dr. Sebi's early life is not widely documented, and he was a self-taught healer with no formal medical training. He claimed to have learned about herbal medicine and healing from his grandmother in Honduras. According to his own accounts, he migrated to the United States in the 1960s and began practicing alternative medicine and offering dietary advice to clients. This marked the beginning of his journey as a holistic healer.

The Dr. Sebi Method

Dr. Sebi's approach to health and healing was based on the belief that many diseases and health problems were the result of mucus buildup in the body, which he referred to as "intracellular mucus." He claimed that this mucus accumulation was primarily caused by an acidic diet and the consumption of unnatural, processed foods, as well as by the use of synthetic medications and drugs.

Dr. Sebi's dietary recommendations were centered around a strict plant-based, alkaline diet. He believed that an alkaline diet could help take out mucus from the body, thereby allowing the body to heal itself naturally. His dietary guidelines included the avoidance of:

1. **Animal products:** Dr. Sebi advocated for a vegan diet, which excluded all animal-based foods, comprising meat, dairy, and eggs.

He argued that animal products were acidic and contributed to mucus formation.

2. **Processed foods:** He advised against consuming processed and refined foods, including white flour and sugar, which he believed were harmful to health.

3. **Hybrid fruits and vegetables:** Dr. Sebi claimed that many fruits and vegetables had been genetically modified and hybridized, making them acidic and unsuitable for consumption. He recommended eating only natural, unhybridized varieties.

4. **Stimulants:** Dr. Sebi discouraged the use of caffeine and other stimulants, as he believed they had a negative impact on the body's natural healing processes.

5. **Medications:** He also urged individuals to avoid pharmaceutical medications, suggesting that they suppressed the body's ability to heal itself.

In contrast, he promoted the consumption of alkaline foods, including whole grains, seeds, nuts, and certain fruits and vegetables. Dr. Sebi was particularly known for his advocacy of the consumption of sea moss (also known as Irish moss), a type of red algae that he claimed had numerous health benefits.

Controversy and Legal Issues
Dr. Sebi's unorthodox approach to health and healing led to significant controversy. He attracted a following of people who believed in the efficacy of his methods, but he also faced skepticism and criticism from the mainstream medical community and regulatory authorities.

One of the key controversies surrounding Dr. Sebi was his claims of being able to cure serious diseases, including cancer and HIV/AIDS, through his dietary recommendations and herbal treatments. Such claims were not substantiated by scientific evidence and were met with skepticism by medical professionals and institutions. In fact, the medical community raised concerns about the potential harm caused by people discontinuing conventional medical treatments in favor of Dr. Sebi's methods.

Dr. Sebi's products, like herbal supplements and tonics, were marketed as part of his healing regimen. However, these products were not approved by the U.S. Food & Drug Administration (FDA), and he faced legal troubles related to their sale and promotion. In 1987, Dr. Sebi was charged with practicing medicine without a license, and his products were labeled as fraudulent by the New York Attorney General's office.

Despite these legal challenges and the lack of scientific validation for his methods, Dr. Sebi continued to promote his dietary recommendations and products, maintaining a loyal following of supporters.

Legacy and Influence
Dr. Sebi's legacy is marked by a polarized reception. His followers believe that he was a visionary healer who offered a natural and holistic approach to health, while critics argue that his claims were unproven and potentially dangerous. His influence can be seen in several areas:

1. **Alternative Medicine:** Dr. Sebi's teachings and dietary recommendations have had a lasting impact on the alternative medicine and natural healing communities. Many people continue to follow his dietary guidelines and use herbal remedies inspired by his work.

2. **Veganism and Plant-Based Diets:** Dr. Sebi's advocacy for a strict vegan diet and the avoidance of processed foods has contributed to the growing popularity of plant-based diets. His emphasis on the alkaline nature of certain foods has also influenced dietary choices among some individuals.

3. **Cultural Impact:** Dr. Sebi's work and teachings have resonated with a primarily African American audience and have become a part of the cultural fabric in some communities. His ideas on natural health and healing are often discussed within the context of Afrocentric movements and cultural awareness.

4. **Online Presence:** Dr. Sebi's message and teachings continue to be disseminated through books, websites, social media, and videos. His influence remains strong in online communities dedicated to holistic health and alternative medicine.

5. **Criticism and Skepticism:** Despite his influence, Dr. Sebi remains a controversial figure, with many skeptics within the medical and scientific communities. His claims of being able to cure serious diseases without scientific validation have drawn criticism and caution from healthcare professionals.

The Foundations of Alkaline and Anti-Inflammatory Diet

In recent years, there has been a growing interest in the concepts of alkaline and anti-inflammatory diets as potential keys to better health and well-being. Both of these dietary approaches are rooted in the idea that the foods we consume can have a significant impact on our body's pH levels and its inflammatory response.

Alkaline Diet Basics

An alkaline diet, also known as the alkaline ash diet or acid-alkaline diet, is based on the principle that the pH level of our body can be influenced by the foods we eat. The pH scale measures acidity or alkalinity, with 7 being neutral, values below 7 indicating acidity, and values above 7 indicating alkalinity. The human body has a tightly regulated pH range, primarily around 7.35 to 7.45, which is slightly alkaline.

The alkaline diet encourages the consumption of foods that promote an alkaline environment in the body, aiming to maintain or restore an ideal pH balance. The key principles of the alkaline diet include:

1. **High Alkaline Foods:** The diet emphasizes the intake of foods that are naturally alkaline or become alkaline-forming during digestion. These foods typically include fruits, vegetables, nuts, seeds, and legumes. Examples of highly alkaline foods are leafy greens, cucumbers, avocados, and almonds.

2. **Low Acidic Foods:** Conversely, the diet discourages the consumption of foods that are acid-forming in the body. Such foods include animal products (meat, dairy), processed foods, sugary items, and grains. These foods are believed to increase acidity in the body and disrupt the pH balance.

3. **Balance:** The goal is to maintain a balanced and varied diet, focusing on alkaline foods while reducing acidic foods. Achieving this balance is thought to support overall health and well-being.

Potential Benefits of an Alkaline Diet

Proponents of the alkaline diet claim that it can offer several health benefits:

1. **Improved Bone Health:** Some research suggests that an alkaline diet may help protect bone health by reducing the loss of calcium from bones. This is because when the body is in an acidic state, it may leach calcium from bones to neutralize the acidity.

2. **Weight Management:** An alkaline diet often promotes the consumption of whole, unprocessed foods, which can lead to weight loss and better weight management. It may also help reduce the risk of obesity-related health issues.

3. **Reduced Inflammation:** Alkaline foods tend to be rich in antioxidants, which can combat inflammation. A diet that minimizes inflammation may reduce the risk of chronic diseases, like heart disease and cancer.

4. **Better Digestive Health:** The diet encourages the consumption of fiber-rich foods, which can improve digestive health and reduce the risk of gastrointestinal issues.

5. **Improved Energy Levels:** Advocates of the diet claim that it can lead to increased energy & vitality due to the elimination of processed and sugary foods.

It's essential to note that while these potential benefits sound promising, scientific research on the alkaline diet is limited and has not conclusively established its effectiveness in preventing or treating diseases. Additionally, the body has natural buffering systems to maintain pH balance, and it is challenging to significantly alter the body's overall pH through diet alone.

Anti-Inflammatory Diet Basics
The concept of an anti-inflammatory diet revolves around the notion that specific foods can either encourage or diminish inflammation in the body.

Chronic inflammation is thought to play a role in the development of many chronic diseases, including heart disease, diabetes, and some cancers. The anti-inflammatory diet focuses on consuming foods that have anti-inflammatory properties and avoiding those that may trigger or exacerbate inflammation.

The key principles of an anti-inflammatory diet include:

1. **High Antioxidant Foods:** Foods rich in antioxidants, like fruits and vegetables, are emphasized. These antioxidants can help combat oxidative stress and reduce inflammation.

2. **Omega-3 Fatty Acids:** Foods that contain omega-3 fatty acids, like fatty fish (e.g., salmon, mackerel, sardines), flaxseeds, and walnuts, are encouraged. Omega-3s have anti-inflammatory properties.

3. **Whole Grains:** Whole grains like quinoa, brown rice, and oats are preferred over refined grains. Whole grains are less likely to trigger inflammation.

4. **Healthy Fats:** Foods with healthy fats, including olive oil, avocados, and nuts, are included in the diet. These fats are associated with reduced inflammation.

5. **Limited Sugar and Processed Foods:** High sugar intake and processed foods can promote inflammation. The anti-inflammatory diet minimizes these foods.

6. **Spices and Herbs:** Certain spices and herbs, like turmeric, ginger & garlic, are known for their anti-inflammatory properties and are often used in this diet.

Potential Benefits of an Anti-Inflammatory Diet
The anti-inflammatory diet is associated with several potential health benefits:

1. **Reduced Risk of Chronic Diseases:** By reducing chronic inflammation, this diet may lower the risk of conditions like heart disease, type 2 diabetes, and certain cancers.

2. **Improved Heart Health:** The emphasis on healthy fats, whole grains, and antioxidants can contribute to better heart health by reducing the risk factors associated with cardiovascular disease.

3. **Joint Health:** Individuals with inflammatory joint conditions like rheumatoid arthritis may experience symptom relief through an anti-inflammatory diet.

4. **Gut Health:** The diet's focus on whole, unprocessed foods and fiber can promote a healthy gut microbiome, which is linked to overall well-being.

5. **Weight Management:** An anti-inflammatory diet's emphasis on whole, nutrient-dense foods can support weight management and reduce obesity-related inflammation.

It's essential to understand that while an anti-inflammatory diet can have numerous health benefits, it is not a cure-all, and its effectiveness may vary from person to person. It is also essential to maintain a balanced and varied diet, as overly restrictive diets can lead to nutritional deficiencies.

Alkaline vs. Anti-Inflammatory Diets
While both alkaline and anti-inflammatory diets share some common elements, they have distinct emphases and objectives:

1. **pH vs. Inflammation:** The primary focus of the alkaline diet is to balance the body's pH levels. It is rooted in the belief that maintaining an alkaline state is essential for good health. In contrast, the anti-inflammatory diet revolves around reducing inflammation as a means to improve health.

2. **Food Categories:** The alkaline diet categorizes foods as either alkaline or acidic, with an emphasis on pH balance. The anti-inflammatory diet categorizes foods based on their potential to either promote or reduce inflammation.

3. **Specific Foods:** The alkaline diet places particular emphasis on avoiding acidic foods, like meat & dairy, and consuming alkaline-forming foods. The anti-inflammatory diet focuses on a broader range of foods that have demonstrated anti-inflammatory properties, like fruits, vegetables, and omega-3 fatty acids.

4. **Balance:** An alkaline diet aims to establish a pH balance by focusing on the proportion of alkaline and acidic foods consumed. The anti-inflammatory diet emphasizes reducing inflammation but does not prescribe specific pH levels.

5. **Flexibility:** The anti-inflammatory diet is more flexible and adaptable to individual dietary preferences and restrictions. It encourages a variety of nutrient-dense foods that can be incorporated into different cultural and culinary traditions.

6. **Scientific Evidence:** The anti-inflammatory diet has a stronger scientific basis, with numerous studies supporting the health benefits of its key principles. The alkaline diet, on the other hand, lacks substantial scientific evidence to confirm its claims.

Incorporating Both Principles

It's worth noting that there can be overlap between the two dietary approaches, and some individuals choose to incorporate elements of both diets into their eating habits. For example, someone might follow an anti-inflammatory diet while also paying attention to the alkalinity or acidity of certain foods they consume.

Here are some tips on how to incorporate elements of both diets into your eating habits:

1. **Prioritize Plant-Based Foods:** Both diets encourage the consumption of a variety of fruits and vegetables, which are rich in antioxidants and tend to be alkaline-forming. Make plant-based foods a central part of your diet.

2. **Include Healthy Fats:** Foods like avocados, nuts, and olive oil are recommended in both diets. Inflammation can be reduced and general health can be supported with the help of these beneficial fats.

3. **Limit Processed Foods:** Both diets discourage processed and sugary foods. Reducing your intake of these items can have a positive impact on your health.

4. **Stay Hydrated:** Maintaining a proper pH balance requires adequate hydration, which can be achieved by consuming water and herbal teas.

5. **Pay Attention to Omega-3s:** Include omega-3-rich foods like fatty fish, flaxseeds & and chia seeds in your diet to reduce inflammation and support overall well-being.

6. **Incorporate Anti-Inflammatory Spices:** Spices like turmeric, ginger, and garlic are not only anti-inflammatory but are often considered alkaline-forming as well. Use them in your cooking for added flavor and health benefits.

7. **Listen to Your Body:** Because each person is distinctive, strategies that work well for one person might not be appropriate for others. Take note to how your body reacts to the various foods you eat, and make adjustments to your diet as necessary.

Chapter 1:

Unveiling the Alkaline Elixir

In the first chapter of our journey into the world of Dr. Sebi's teachings, we will explore the foundational principles of the Alkaline Diet, a dietary approach that echoes the wisdom of the ages. This ancient wisdom, often overlooked in the hustle and bustle of modern life, holds the key to rejuvenating our bodies, minds, and spirits. Let's delve into the core principles and profound benefits of the Alkaline Diet.

Understanding Body pH

pH, which stands for "potential of hydrogen," is a measurement of the acidity or alkalinity of a substance. It is expressed on a scale from 0 - 14, with 0 being highly acidic, 14 highly alkaline, and 7 being neutral. The concept of pH is essential in various scientific disciplines, including chemistry, biology, and medicine. In the context of the human body, maintaining an appropriate pH level is crucial for overall health and well-being.

The pH Scale
Because the pH scale is a logarithmic scale, each full number on the scale signifies a tenfold change in the degree to which acidity or alkalinity has been increased or decreased. To illustrate, a substance with a pH of 3 is tenfold more acidic compared to one with a pH of 4. Likewise, a substance with a pH of 9 is tenfold more alkaline than a substance with a pH of 8.

- pH 0-6: Acidic

- pH 7: Neutral
- pH 8-14: Alkaline (or basic)

In the human body, different parts and fluids have specific pH values to maintain their functions. For example:

1. **Blood:** Blood pH is tightly regulated within a narrow range, typically between 7.35 and 7.45. Deviations from this range can be life-threatening.

2. **Stomach Acid:** The stomach's acidic environment is crucial for the digestion of food and the destruction of harmful microorganisms. Stomach acid has a pH of 1.5 - 3.5.

3. **Urine:** Urine pH can vary, but it is generally slightly acidic, with a range of 4.5 to 8.0.

4. **Skin:** The pH of the skin varies depending on its location and the individual, but it is typically slightly acidic, around 5.5.

pH Regulation in the Body
Maintaining the body's pH within a narrow and specific range is essential for proper functioning. The body has several mechanisms to regulate pH, including:

1. **Buffer Systems:** Buffer systems in the blood and body fluids consist of a combination of weak acids and bases that help resist changes in pH. They can absorb or release hydrogen ions to maintain pH stability.

2. **Respiratory System:** The levels of carbon dioxide (CO_2) in the blood are controlled by the respiratory system, which is one of the factors that contributes to pH regulation. When there is a rise in CO_2 levels, carbonic acid is formed, which can cause the pH to

drop. The body is able to eliminate excess CO_2 and elevate pH by modifying the rate at which it breathes as well as the depth to which it breathes.

3. **Renal System:** The kidneys play a significant role in regulating pH. They can excrete hydrogen ions to lower pH or reabsorb bicarbonate ions to raise pH. The renal system's regulation is slower than that of the respiratory system but is crucial for maintaining pH over the long term.

4. **Diet and Metabolism:** The foods we eat can impact the body's pH. For example, the breakdown of certain nutrients can result in the production of acids or bases. The body can also regulate pH through the excretion of excess acid or base in urine.

Acidosis and Alkalosis
When the body's pH falls outside the normal range, it can lead to two primary conditions: acidosis and alkalosis.

Acidosis: Acidosis occurs when the blood becomes too acidic, typically with a pH below 7.35. It can result from an excess of hydrogen ions or a decrease in bicarbonate ions. Acidosis can be caused by various factors, including kidney dysfunction, respiratory problems, metabolic disorders, or the ingestion of acidic substances.

- **Respiratory Acidosis:** This takes place when the respiratory system is unable to expel a sufficient amount of carbon dioxide, leading to an increase in carbonic acid in the blood.
- **Metabolic Acidosis:** This can result from the accumulation of metabolic acids due to conditions like diabetic ketoacidosis, lactic acidosis, or kidney dysfunction.

Alkalosis: Alkalosis occurs when the blood becomes too alkaline, typically with a pH above 7.45. It can be caused by a loss of hydrogen ions or an increase in bicarbonate ions. Alkalosis can result from factors like hyperventilation, vomiting, or the excessive use of antacids.

- **Respiratory Alkalosis:** It occurs when the respiratory system eliminates too much carbon dioxide, reducing carbonic acid levels in the blood.
- **Metabolic Alkalosis:** This can result from the loss of acids through conditions like excessive vomiting, certain medications, or electrolyte imbalances.

pH and Health
The body's pH balance plays a critical role in health, and maintaining the appropriate pH in different bodily fluids is essential for various physiological processes. Here are some key ways in which pH is linked to health:

1. **Blood pH:** Maintaining blood pH within the narrow range of 7.35 - 7.45 is crucial for normal cellular function. Even slight deviations from this range can disrupt enzymatic activity, protein structure, and overall metabolic processes. Acidosis and alkalosis can have serious health consequences, affecting the central nervous system, the cardiovascular system, and other organ systems.

2. **Stomach Acid:** The highly acidic environment in the stomach, with a pH of 1.5 to 3.5, is necessary for the digestion of food and the activation of digestive enzymes. It also plays a role in protecting against harmful bacteria and pathogens that may enter the body through food and drink.

3. **Digestion and Nutrient Absorption:** The pH of various parts of the digestive tract, including the stomach and small intestine,

influences the digestion and absorption of nutrients. Proper pH levels in these regions are essential for breaking down food and extracting essential vitamins and minerals.

4. **Skin pH:** The skin's slightly acidic pH of around 5.5 helps maintain the skin's barrier function and prevents the growth of harmful microorganisms. Changes in skin pH can lead to skin conditions and infections.

5. **Urine pH:** The pH of urine can provide insights into various health conditions. For example, highly acidic urine may indicate metabolic problems or dehydration, while highly alkaline urine may be a sign of certain urinary tract issues or a diet rich in alkaline foods.

6. **Bone Health:** Some proponents of the alkaline diet believe that an overly acidic diet may lead to calcium loss from bones, contributing to osteoporosis.

7. **Cancer and pH:** There is a popular but scientifically unproven theory that suggests an alkaline diet can prevent or treat cancer by creating an unfavorable environment for cancer cells. This theory lacks empirical support from clinical trials, and cancer treatment should always be guided by established medical practices.

Diet and Body pH

Diet can influence the body's pH, but it's essential to understand the nuances of how this works. While certain foods can have an impact on the pH of bodily fluids like urine, they have limited direct influence on blood pH. Blood pH is tightly regulated by the body, and it does not fluctuate significantly in response to dietary changes.

However, dietary choices can affect the pH of urine. For example, consuming foods high in acid-forming compounds, like animal proteins and processed foods, may result in more acidic urine. Conversely, diets rich in fruits and vegetables, which are alkaline-forming, may lead to more alkaline urine. But it's essential to remember that urine pH is not necessarily indicative of overall health, and it can vary throughout the day.

Body pH and Exercise
Physical activity can influence body pH, particularly during intense exercise. Here's how:

1. **Lactic Acid Buildup:** During strenuous exercise, lactic acid can accumulate in muscles and the bloodstream. This can lead to a temporary decrease in pH and cause muscle fatigue and soreness. However, the body's buffer systems and the respiratory system work to restore pH to normal levels once exercise ceases.

2. **Respiratory Acidosis:** Very intense exercise can lead to increased CO_2 production and a temporary drop in pH, resulting in respiratory acidosis. The body compensates by increasing ventilation to eliminate excess CO_2, which helps restore normal pH levels.

3. **Hydration:** Dehydration can lead to a concentration of acids in the bloodstream, potentially lowering pH. Staying well-hydrated is essential for maintaining a stable pH during exercise.

Overall, regular exercise is associated with improved health and is not typically a direct cause of chronic pH imbalances. The body's regulatory systems help maintain pH equilibrium, and any exercise-induced fluctuations are generally temporary and part of the body's natural response to physical exertion.

The Significance of Alkalinity

Alkalinity, often referred to in the context of body pH, is a concept that has gained significant attention in recent years. The idea is rooted in the belief that maintaining an alkaline environment in the body can promote better health and well-being.

Understanding Alkalinity

Alkalinity, in the context of body pH, refers to the state of being slightly alkaline or basic. The pH scale, spanning from 0 (indicating high acidity) to 14 (indicating high alkalinity), presents as a measure for determining the acidity or alkalinity of a substance. In this scale, a pH of 7 is considered neutral. The human body has a pH range within which it functions optimally, primarily around 7.35 to 7.45, making it slightly alkaline.

The significance of alkalinity in the body relates to maintaining this narrow pH range in various bodily fluids, particularly the blood. Deviations from this range can have adverse effects on health. For example, if the blood becomes too acidic (a condition known as acidosis), it can interfere with enzymatic activity, protein structure, and overall metabolic processes. Conversely, if the blood becomes too alkaline (alkalosis), it can also disrupt normal bodily functions.

The Role of Alkalinity in the Body

Alkalinity plays a crucial role in the body and is involved in several physiological processes. Here are some key areas where alkalinity is significant:

1. **Blood pH Balance:** Maintaining the slightly alkaline pH of the blood is essential for normal cellular function. The body has robust mechanisms for regulating blood pH and preventing it from becoming too acidic or too alkaline.

2. **Digestive Health:** The pH of the stomach is highly acidic, typically ranging from 1.5 to 3.5. This acidity is necessary for the digestion of food and the activation of digestive enzymes. It also presents as a defense mechanism against harmful microorganisms and pathogens that may enter the body through food and drink.

3. **Enzyme Function:** Many enzymes in the body are sensitive to changes in pH. Maintaining an appropriate pH is crucial for the efficiency of enzymatic reactions that are vital for metabolism, energy production, and other cellular processes.

4. **Mineral Absorption:** The pH of various parts of the digestive tract, like the small intestine, influences the absorption of minerals. Proper pH levels in these regions are necessary for breaking down food and extracting essential vitamins and minerals.

5. **Skin Barrier Function:** The skin's slightly acidic pH, typically around 5.5, helps maintain its barrier function and protects against harmful microorganisms. Changes in skin pH can lead to skin conditions and infections.

6. **Urinary pH:** Urine pH can provide insights into various health conditions. Highly acidic urine may indicate metabolic

problems or dehydration, while highly alkaline urine may be a sign of urinary tract issues or a diet rich in alkaline foods.

Incorporating Alkalinity into a Balanced Diet
While the scientific support for the alkaline diet's specific claims is limited, there is value in incorporating alkaline-forming foods into a balanced and healthy diet. Here are some tips on how to do so:

1. **Prioritize Plant-Based Foods:** Both the alkaline diet and general health guidelines emphasize the consumption of a variety of fruits & vegetables. These foods are high in vitamins, antioxidants, and minerals and tend to be alkaline-forming. Make plant-based foods a central part of your diet.

2. **Include Healthy Fats:** Foods like avocados, nuts, and olive oil are recommended in both the alkaline diet and a balanced diet. These healthy fats can support overall health.

3. **Limit Processed Foods:** Both the alkaline diet and general health guidelines discourage processed and sugary foods. Reducing your intake of these items can have a positive impact on your health.

4. **Stay Hydrated:** Ensuring adequate hydration is crucial for preserving a balanced pH. Consuming water and herbal teas can assist in maintaining your hydration levels.

5. **Incorporate Anti-Inflammatory Spices:** Spices like turmeric, ginger, and garlic are not only anti-inflammatory but are often considered alkaline-forming as well. Use them in your cooking for added flavor and health benefits.

6. **Listen to Your Body:** Because each person is unique, strategies that work well for one person might not be appropriate for others. Pay attention to how your body reacts to the various foods you eat, and make adjustments to your diet as necessary.

The Mucus Link to Diseases

Mucus, a viscous and slimy substance produced by the body's mucous membranes, plays an essential role in protecting and maintaining the health of various organs and tissues. It lines the respiratory, digestive, and reproductive tracts, serving as a defense mechanism against pathogens, irritants, and injury. However, an imbalance or overproduction of mucus can be linked to various diseases & health conditions.

The Role of Mucus in the Body
Mucus, also known as phlegm when it is produced in the respiratory system, is a complex secretion composed of water, proteins, lipids, and various other compounds. It presents several critical functions in the body, including:

1. **Protection:** Mucus acts as a physical barrier that traps and immobilizes foreign particles, including dust, bacteria, viruses, and other pathogens. This protective function helps prevent these invaders from entering and infecting the body.

2. **Moisturization:** Mucus presents to maintain the moisture of mucous membrane surfaces and prevents them from drying out. This is especially essential in the respiratory and digestive tracts to facilitate the movement of cilia and the transit of food and air.

3. **Immune Defense:** Mucus contains immune molecules and cells that can help neutralize and destroy pathogens. It plays a role in the innate immune response, which is the body's first line of defense against infections.

4. **Transport:** Mucus aids in the movement of substances through various parts of the body. For example, in the respiratory tract, mucus helps to transport trapped particles out of the lungs.

Diseases and Conditions Associated with Mucus
While mucus is essential for maintaining health, an imbalance in its production or composition can contribute to a range of diseases & health conditions. Here are some examples:

Respiratory Conditions

- **Cystic Fibrosis:** It is a hereditary condition that leads to the creation of dense, adhesive mucus in the respiratory and digestive systems. This atypical mucus can block the airways, causing breathing difficulties and heightening the susceptibility to lung infections.
- **Chronic Obstructive Pulmonary Disease (COPD):** It includes conditions like chronic bronchitis and emphysema, characterized by chronic inflammation of the airways. In these diseases, increased mucus production and changes in mucus composition contribute to airway obstruction and breathing difficulties.
- **Asthma:** Asthma is a persistent respiratory ailment marked by airway inflammation and heightened mucus production. This surplus mucus can block the air passages, resulting in symptoms like wheezing, coughing, and breathlessness.

Upper Respiratory Infections

- **Common Cold:** Viral infections, like the common cold, can trigger an overproduction of mucus in the upper respiratory tract, causing symptoms like a congested or runny nose.
- **Sinusitis:** Inflammation of the sinuses can cause mucus to become thick and block the sinuses, leading to sinusitis. This condition can result in facial pain, pressure, and nasal congestion.

Gastrointestinal Conditions

- **Gastroesophageal Reflux Disease (GERD):** In cases of GERD (Gastroesophageal Reflux Disease), stomach acid has the potential to reflux into the esophagus, resulting in irritation and inflammation. The body may produce excess mucus in response to protect the esophageal lining.
- **Inflammatory Bowel Disease (IBD):** Conditions like Crohn's disease and ulcerative colitis are defined by persistent inflammation of the digestive tract. This inflammation can lead to elevated mucus production, which in turn can contribute to symptoms like diarrhea and abdominal pain.

Reproductive Health

- **Cervical Mucus Changes:** Changes in cervical mucus can be indicative of hormonal imbalances or infections. Abnormal cervical mucus can affect fertility and may be linked to conditions like polycystic ovary syndrome (PCOS).
  - **Allergies:** Allergic reactions to environmental allergens, like pollen, dust mites, or pet dander, can lead to an increased production of mucus in the respiratory system. This can result in symptoms like sneezing, a runny or stuffy nose, and itchy, watery eyes.

o **Infections:** Infections in various parts of the body, like the respiratory, urinary, or reproductive tracts, can lead to increased mucus production as the body's defense mechanism against pathogens.

Chronic Mucus Production and Inflammation

Chronic mucus production can be a response to persistent inflammation in the body. While inflammation is a natural component of the body's immune response, persistent inflammation can lead to alterations in both the production and composition of mucus. This, in turn, can contribute to the development and progression of various diseases.

For example, in chronic respiratory conditions like COPD and asthma, ongoing inflammation of the airways leads to increased mucus production and changes in the structure of mucus, making it more difficult to clear from the airways. This chronic mucus production contributes to airway obstruction and worsens the conditions.

Inflammatory bowel diseases like Crohn's disease and ulcerative colitis are characterized by persistent inflammation in the digestive tract, which can lead to increased mucus production and changes in mucus composition. This contributes to the gastrointestinal symptoms associated with these conditions.

Mucus as a Diagnostic Tool

In some cases, analyzing the characteristics of mucus can be a valuable diagnostic tool. For example:

1. **Sputum Analysis:** For respiratory illnesses, examining the properties of sputum (the phlegm expelled from the lungs) can aid in pinpointing the root cause of an individual's symptoms. For example, the color, thickness, and presence of blood in sputum can provide essential diagnostic information.

2. **Cervical Mucus Examination:** Changes in cervical mucus can be assessed as part of fertility awareness methods. The consistency and appearance of cervical mucus can help individuals track their menstrual cycle and identify fertile periods.

3. **Stool Analysis:** In gastrointestinal disorders, examining the characteristics of stool, including the presence of mucus, can provide insights into digestive health and potential conditions like infections, inflammation, or malabsorption.

Treatment and Management
The management of diseases and conditions related to mucus often involves addressing the underlying cause and relieving symptoms. Treatment options may include:

1. **Medications:** In respiratory conditions, medications like bronchodilators, corticosteroids, and mucolytics may be prescribed to alleviate symptoms and reduce mucus production.

2. **Lifestyle Modifications:** For conditions related to allergies, lifestyle modifications like allergen avoidance, the use of air purifiers, and changes in dietary habits may help reduce symptoms.

3. **Dietary Changes:** In gastrointestinal conditions, dietary adjustments may be recommended to alleviate symptoms and support digestive health.

4. **Physical Therapy:** Chest physical therapy, which includes techniques to help clear mucus from the airways, is often used in the treatment of respiratory conditions.

5. **Antibiotics:** In the case of infections, antibiotics may be prescribed to target the underlying pathogen.

6. **Surgical Interventions:** In certain instances, surgical interventions may be required to manage chronic conditions or complications associated with mucus production.

Chapter 2:

The Sebian Scripture

In this chapter, we delve into the heart of Dr. Sebi's teachings and philosophy, uncovering his curated list of approved and non-approved foods that form the cornerstone of his approach to wellness. Dr. Sebi's profound understanding of the intricate relationship between diet and disease has paved the way for a comprehensive guide to achieving optimal health through conscious food choices.

Approved and Non-Approved Foods

List of Approved Foods on the Dr. Sebi Diet:
The Dr. Sebi diet included a range of approved foods that adhered to the principles of plant-based, alkaline, and raw eating. These foods were believed to be beneficial for the body and were encouraged for consumption. Some of the approved foods included:

1. **Fruits:** Such as bananas, berries, melons, and citrus fruits like lemons and limes.

2. **Vegetables:** This category encompasses leafy greens like kale and spinach, along with root vegetables like sweet potatoes.

3. **Nuts & Seeds:** Such as almonds, walnuts, and chia seeds.

4. **Grains:** Particularly whole grains like quinoa and wild rice.

5. **Herbal Teas:** Natural herbal teas, like chamomile and ginger tea, were recommended.

6. **Nutritional Supplements:** Dr. Sebi's dietary recommendations often included the use of his own herbal supplements, like the "African Bio-Mineral Balance" compounds.

It's essential to note that the Dr. Sebi diet discouraged the consumption of hybrid foods, which he claimed were unnatural and harmful to the body. Hybrid foods are plants that have been crossbred to create new varieties, like many modern fruits and vegetables. Dr. Sebi believed that hybrid foods disrupted the body's natural healing processes and should be avoided.

List of Non-Approved Foods on the Dr. Sebi Diet:
The Dr. Sebi diet also included a list of non-approved foods, which were believed to be harmful and mucus-forming. These foods were strongly discouraged or even prohibited on the diet. Some of the non-approved foods included:

1. **Animal Products:** All forms of animal products, including meat, dairy, and eggs, were considered detrimental to health and were to be eliminated from the diet.

2. **Processed and Refined Foods:** This category included foods like white sugar, white flour, and processed snacks. Dr. Sebi believed that these foods disrupted the body's natural healing processes.

3. **Hybrid Fruits and Vegetables:** As mentioned earlier, hybrid fruits and vegetables were discouraged because they were considered unnatural and harmful.

4. **Starchy Foods:** Foods high in starch, like bread and white potatoes, were also considered mucus-forming and were to be avoided.

5. **Caffeine:** Dr. Sebi discouraged the consumption of caffeinated beverages like coffee and tea.

6. **Alcohol:** Alcoholic beverages were considered harmful to the body and were not recommended.

7. **Artificial Sweeteners:** Artificial sweeteners like aspartame were discouraged in favor of natural sweeteners like agave nectar.

The Core Principles of Dr. Sebi's Diet

Dr. Sebi, also known as Alfredo Darrington Bowman, was a controversial Honduran herbalist and self-proclaimed healer known for promoting a specific dietary philosophy aimed at achieving optimal health and well-being. Dr. Sebi's diet, often referred to as the Dr. Sebi nutritional guide, was based on the idea that a plant-based, alkaline diet could help the body heal and rejuvenate itself. Through his teachings, Dr. Sebi emphasized the importance of consuming natural, unprocessed foods to detoxify the body and promote overall wellness.

1. **Plant-Based Nutrition**

One of the fundamental principles of Dr. Sebi's diet is the emphasis on plant-based nutrition. Dr. Sebi promoted the consumption of a diverse range of fresh, natural, and organic plant-based foods, which encompassed fruits, vegetables, nuts, seeds, and whole grains. He held the belief that a plant-centered diet could offer the essential nutrients required for maintaining excellent health while avoiding the adverse effects often linked to the consumption of animal products.

According to Dr. Sebi, plant-based foods are easier for the body to digest and assimilate, leading to improved overall health. He often recommended the consumption of a diverse range of fruits and vegetables, encouraging individuals to incorporate them into their daily meals to promote wellness and vitality.

2. Alkaline Approach

Dr. Sebi's diet heavily promoted the consumption of alkaline foods and beverages while discouraging the intake of acidic foods. He claimed that an alkaline-rich diet could help maintain the body's pH balance and prevent the development of various illnesses and diseases.

According to Dr. Sebi, acidic foods, like processed foods, refined sugars, and animal products, could disrupt the body's natural pH balance and contribute to the accumulation of mucus, inflammation, and various health issues. On the other hand, he believed that alkaline foods, including many fruits and vegetables, could help neutralize acidity and create a more balanced and harmonious internal environment.

3. Elimination of Processed and Hybrid Foods

Dr. Sebi's dietary philosophy involved the complete elimination of processed and hybrid foods from one's diet. He asserted that processed and genetically modified foods contained harmful substances and additives that could disrupt the body's natural healing processes and contribute to the development of chronic diseases.

Furthermore, Dr. Sebi warned against the consumption of hybrid fruits and vegetables, claiming that they lacked the essential nutrients found in their natural, unaltered counterparts. He advocated for the consumption of organic, non-hybrid, and non-GMO foods to ensure that the body received the maximum nutritional benefits without any harmful additives or modifications.

4. Raw and Uncooked Foods

Dr. Sebi encouraged the consumption of raw and uncooked foods, believing that the natural enzymes and nutrients present in these foods were crucial for supporting the body's overall health and vitality. He claimed that cooking food at high temperatures destroyed essential nutrients and enzymes, making it less beneficial for the body.

According to Dr. Sebi, raw and uncooked foods retained their natural vitality and were easier for the body to digest and absorb. He often recommended the consumption of raw fruits and vegetables, nuts, seeds, and grains to maximize the intake of essential nutrients and enzymes necessary for promoting optimal health.

5. Herbal Supplements

In addition to dietary recommendations, Dr. Sebi also advocated for the use of specific herbal supplements and botanical remedies to support the body's natural healing processes. He held the belief that specific herbs and plants harbored potent healing properties capable of aiding in body detoxification, enhancing the immune system, and reinstating equilibrium within various bodily systems.

Dr. Sebi frequently created and endorsed his own range of herbal supplements, asserting that they could address particular health issues and enhance overall health. These herbal supplements were often designed to work synergistically with the dietary principles of the Dr. Sebi nutritional guide, aiming to provide comprehensive support for the body's natural healing mechanisms.

6. Detoxification and Cellular Health

Detoxification was a central theme in Dr. Sebi's teachings, as he believed that the body needed to regularly eliminate toxins and waste products to maintain optimal health. He frequently stressed the need of ingesting foods that are high in cleaning properties and nutrients in order to encourage the natural detoxification processes of the body and to enhance cellular health.

Dr. Sebi encouraged the consumption of foods with natural detoxifying properties, like leafy greens, cruciferous vegetables, and specific herbs and spices known for their cleansing and purifying effects. He believed that regular detoxification could help improve overall well-being and reduce the risk of various chronic diseases and health complications.

7. Hydration and Alkaline Water

Proper hydration was considered essential in Dr. Sebi's dietary approach. He recommended the consumption of alkaline water, which he believed could help balance the body's pH levels and support overall health. Alkaline water was thought to have a higher pH level than regular water, making it more alkaline and, according to Dr. Sebi, more beneficial for the body.

Dr. Sebi encouraged individuals to prioritize the consumption of alkaline water and herbal teas to support hydration and overall well-being. He often recommended the use of natural and organic beverages over sugary or artificially flavored drinks to avoid the negative effects associated with excessive sugar and additives.

Transitioning to an Alkaline Diet

If you're interested in transitioning to an alkaline diet, here are some steps to help you get started:

1. Educate Yourself

Before making any dietary changes, it's essential to understand the basic principles of the alkaline diet. Learn about the difference between alkaline-forming and acid-forming foods, and familiarize yourself with the pH values of common foods. This knowledge will guide your food choices.

2. Assess Your Current Diet

Take a close look at your current eating habits. Identify the foods you consume regularly and determine whether they are alkaline-forming or acid-forming. This self-assessment will give you insights into how far you need to transition toward an alkaline diet.

3. Set Realistic Goals

Transitioning to a new diet can be challenging, so it's essential to set realistic and achievable goals. You might start by gradually incorporating more alkaline foods into your meals and reducing the intake of acidic foods.

4. Increase Alkaline Foods

Begin to include more alkaline-forming foods in your diet. Here are some examples:

- Fruits: Relish a variety of fresh fruits, like berries, apples, pears, and citrus fruits.
- Vegetables: Make sure your plate is filled with colorful vegetables like leafy greens, broccoli, carrots, and bell peppers.
- Nuts and Seeds: Incorporate almonds, walnuts, chia seeds, and flaxseeds into your meals and snacks.
- Legumes: Include beans, lentils, and chickpeas to your diet for plant-based protein.
- Whole Grains: Choose whole grains like quinoa, brown rice, and oats for a healthier carbohydrate source.

5. Decrease Acidic Foods

Gradually reduce the consumption of acid-forming foods. This may include:

- Animal Products: Cut back on meat, dairy, and eggs. Consider plant-based alternatives if you're transitioning to a vegan or vegetarian diet.
- Processed Foods: Limit or eliminate processed and highly refined foods, including sugary snacks, fast food, and packaged convenience meals.
- Sugar and Caffeine: Reduce your intake of sugary foods and beverages, and consider substituting your daily coffee with herbal tea or alkaline water.

6. **Balance Your Meals**

Strive for balanced meals that include a variety of alkaline-forming foods. Consider creating balanced, plant-based dishes, like quinoa salad with mixed vegetables, bean and avocado wraps, or fruit smoothies with added greens.

7. **Stay Hydrated**

Proper hydration is vital for maintaining overall health and pH balance. Alkaline water is often recommended on this diet. You can also include a squeeze of fresh lemon or lime to your water, as these citrus fruits, while acidic in nature, have an alkalizing effect on the body when metabolized.

8. **Plan Your Meals**

Meal planning can be a helpful tool in ensuring that you have access to alkaline foods throughout the week. Prepare and store alkaline-rich foods in advance to make it convenient to follow your dietary goals.

9. **Experiment with Alkaline Recipes**

Explore alkaline recipes to make your meals enjoyable and varied. There are many creative recipes available that cater to the alkaline diet, allowing you to savor the flavors of alkaline foods.

10. **Monitor Your Progress**

Keep a journal of your dietary choices and how you feel as you transition to an alkaline diet. Pay attention to changes in your energy levels, digestion, and overall well-being. This will help you track your progress and make any necessary adjustments.

11. **Consult a Healthcare Professional**

Before implementing substantial alterations to your diet, it is advisable to ask advice from a healthcare professional or a registered dietitian. They can offer tailored recommendations and ensure that your dietary decisions are in harmony with your health objectives and unique requirements.

Chapter 3:

The Anti-Inflammation

Odyssey

In this chapter, we embark on an exploration of the intertwined realms of acidity, inflammation, and the profound impact of the alkaline diet as a beacon of alleviation. We delve into the crucial connections between our body's acidic state, inflammation, and the transformative potential of adopting an alkaline diet. Join us as we unravel the Anti-Inflammation Odyssey.

The Importance of Detoxification

Detoxification, often referred to as detox for short, is a process by which the body eliminates or neutralizes harmful substances and waste products to maintain health and well-being. While the concept of detoxification has been a topic of discussion and practice for centuries, its importance in modern times has gained significant attention.

Understanding Detoxification
Detoxification is a fundamental and continuous physiological process that takes place in the human body. It involves the removal of toxins, waste products, and harmful substances from various organs and systems, allowing the body to function efficiently and maintain its balance. This natural process is primarily carried out by the liver, kidneys, lungs, skin, and the lymphatic system.

Here's a breakdown of the key organs involved in detoxification:

1. **Liver:** The liver plays a central role in detoxification. It processes and neutralizes toxins, making them easier for the body to eliminate. The liver is also responsible for producing enzymes and other substances that aid in the detoxification process.

2. **Kidneys:** The kidneys filter waste products and toxins from the blood, which are then excreted as urine.

3. **Lungs:** The lungs eliminate gaseous waste products, like carbon dioxide, during respiration.

4. **Skin:** The skin presents as the body's largest organ of elimination. It releases waste products and toxins through sweat.

5. **Lymphatic System:** The lymphatic system, which includes lymph nodes and vessels, helps transport and filter waste products and toxins from various tissues and organs.

Why Detoxification is Important
The importance of detoxification stems from the fact that our modern environment exposes us to a wide range of toxins and harmful substances. These toxins can come from various sources, including:

- **Environmental Toxins:** Pollutants in the air and water, pesticides, heavy metals, & chemicals in household products can introduce toxins into our bodies.
- **Diet:** Consuming processed and highly refined foods, artificial additives, and excessive sugar and caffeine can burden the body with toxins.
- **Medications:** Some medications, when used over extended periods, may lead to the accumulation of toxins in the body.

- **Stress:** Chronic stress can impact the body's detoxification systems and increase the production of stress hormones, potentially leading to negative health effects.
- **Alcohol & Tobacco:** The consumption of alcohol and tobacco can introduce toxins into the body, impacting the liver, lungs, and other organs.

The accumulation of these toxins can lead to various health issues and contribute to chronic conditions, like liver disease, kidney problems, digestive disorders, and skin problems. Detoxification is essential for maintaining the body's natural balance and reducing the risk of toxin-related health problems.

The Benefits of Detoxification
A well-functioning detoxification process offers numerous benefits for overall health and well-being:

1. **Improved Energy and Vitality:** Detoxification can lead to increased energy levels and improved vitality, as the body is better equipped to carry out its functions without the burden of excess toxins.

2. **Clearer Skin:** Effective detoxification can lead to healthier, clearer skin by eliminating toxins that can contribute to skin problems.

3. **Better Digestion:** A cleaner gastrointestinal system can lead to improved digestion & better absorption of nutrients.

4. **Weight Management:** Detoxification can help with weight loss and weight management by eliminating excess waste and promoting a healthier metabolism.

5. **Enhanced Immune Function:** A detoxified body is more capable of fighting off infections and illnesses, leading to better immune function.

6. **Reduced Inflammation:** Detoxification could aid in decreasing chronic inflammation, which is a common factor in many diseases and health issues.

7. **Improved Mental Clarity:** Some people report enhanced mental clarity, focus, and reduced brain fog after detoxification.

Natural Detox Techniques

Detoxification, often referred to as detox, is the process of removing toxins & waste products from the body to support overall health and well-being. While there are various methods for detoxification, including dietary changes and supplements, many people prefer natural detox techniques. These methods focus on using the body's innate detoxification systems, like the , skin, liver, kidneys and lungs, to eliminate harmful substances.

1. **Hydration**

Staying well-hydrated is one of the most fundamental natural detox techniques. Water is essential for flushing waste products and toxins out of the body through urine, sweat, and respiration. Adequate hydration facilitates the operation of the kidneys, which play a crucial role in filtering waste from the bloodstream.

Tips for proper hydration:

- Strive to consume a minimum of eight 8-ounce glasses of water daily, following the "8x8" rule, or adjust your intake as needed based on your level of physical activity and the climate you are in.

- Consider carrying a reusable water bottle to help you track and maintain your daily water intake.
- Enhance the detoxifying effect of water by adding a squeeze of fresh lemon or a few slices of cucumber to your water. Both lemon and cucumber have natural detoxifying properties.

2. Whole Foods Diet

A whole foods diet is another essential natural detox technique. Eating whole, unprocessed foods, especially those that are rich in fiber and antioxidants, can help support your body's natural detoxification processes. These foods provide essential nutrients while reducing the burden of toxins and harmful substances.

Foods to include in a whole foods diet:

- **Fruits & vegetables:** Opt for a diverse selection of colorful fruits & vegetables to obtain a broad spectrum of vitamins, minerals, and antioxidants.

- **Whole grains:** Opt for whole grains like brown rice, quinoa, and oats over processed grains.
- **Legumes:** Beans, lentils, and chickpeas provide plant-based protein and fiber.
- **Nuts and seeds:** Almonds, walnuts, chia seeds, and flaxseeds are nutritious additions.
- **Lean protein:** If you include animal products, choose lean, organic options and consume them in moderation.

3. Herbal Teas

Herbal teas, like dandelion, milk thistle, ginger, and peppermint, are natural detoxifiers that can support your liver and digestive system. These teas have been used for centuries to aid in the removal of toxins & waste products from the body.

Popular herbal teas for detoxification:

- **Dandelion tea:** These is known for its diuretic properties, which can help take out excess water and toxins from the body. It also supports liver health.
- **Milk thistle tea:** Milk thistle is thought to safeguard the liver and stimulate the renewal of liver cells, rendering it a valuable herb for the process of detoxification.
- **Ginger tea:** Ginger assists in digestion, mitigates inflammation, and can contribute to the removal of waste and toxins from the digestive system.
- **Peppermint tea:** Peppermint tea calms the digestive tract and supports proper digestion, a crucial aspect of the detoxification process.

4. **Exercise**

Regular physical activity is a powerful natural detox technique. Exercise increases circulation, which enhances the removal of waste products and toxins from the body. It also promotes sweating, a natural way for the body to eliminate toxins through the skin.

Types of exercise to support detoxification:

- **Aerobic exercise:** Activities like brisk walking, jogging, cycling, and swimming increase heart rate and circulation, promoting the removal of waste products through sweat & respiration.
- **Strength training:** Building lean muscle mass can boost metabolism and improve overall body function, including detoxification processes.

- **Yoga:** Yoga combines physical postures, deep breathing, and meditation, providing relaxation and stress reduction, which can support detoxification.

5. **Dry Brushing**

Dry brushing is a simple and effective natural detox technique that involves using a dry brush with stiff bristles to gently brush the skin. This technique stimulates the lymphatic system, which helps eliminate waste and toxins from the body.

How to dry brush:

- Start with a dry brush with natural bristles.
- Begin brushing at your feet and move upward, always brushing in the direction of your heart.
- Use long, sweeping motions, and avoid brushing too hard, as the goal is to stimulate, not irritate, the skin.
- Shower or bathe after dry brushing to wash away any dead skin cells and impurities that were loosened during the process.

6. **Sauna and Steam Baths**

Saunas and steam baths can be beneficial natural detox techniques that promote sweating. Sweating is a natural mechanism by which the body expels toxins through the skin. Heat from saunas and steam baths increases circulation and helps the body release waste products.

Considerations when using saunas and steam baths:

- Ensure you stay hydrated before, during, and after the sauna or steam bath to replace lost fluids through sweating.
- Limit the time you spend in a sauna or steam bath to prevent dehydration and overheating.

- If you have underlying health conditions or are taking medications, consult a healthcare professional before using saunas and steam baths.

7. **Deep Breathing Exercises**

These exercises, like diaphragmatic breathing and pranayama from yoga, could aid in decreasing stress and support the body's natural detoxification processes. Stress reduction is essential for overall health, as chronic stress can negatively impact detoxification systems.

How to practice deep breathing:

- Locate a serene and comfortable spot to either sit or recline.
- Inhale deeply through your nose, allowing your diaphragm to expand.
- Exhale slowly and completely through your mouth.
- Repeat this routine for a few mins, concentrating on your breath and releasing stress and tension.

8. **Epsom Salt Baths**

Epsom salt baths can be a relaxing and natural detox technique that supports the removal of toxins from the body. Epsom salt, also recognized as magnesium sulfate, is absorbed through the skin while bathing, delivering magnesium and sulfur, which can assist in the detoxification process.

How to take an Epsom salt bath:

- Fill your bathtub with warm water.
- Incorporate approximately 2 teacups of Epsom salt into the bathwater and stir till dissolved.

- Immerse yourself in the bath for 20-30 mins to enable your body to absorb the Epsom salt.

9. **Intermittent Fasting**

Intermittent fasting refers to an eating regimen that involves alternating between designated intervals of eating and fasting. It can be an effective natural detox technique that allows the digestive system to rest and supports the body's natural cleansing processes.

Common intermittent fasting methods:

- **16/8 method:** This approach entails fasting for 16 hrs and confining your eating to an 8-hour window daily.
- **5:2 method:** In this approach, you consume a regular diet for five days a week and restrict calorie intake to around 500-600 calories on the other two non-consecutive days.
- **Alternate-day fasting:** With this method, you alternate between days of normal eating and days of fasting or consuming very few calories.

10. **Mindfulness and Meditation**

Practicing mindfulness and meditation can reduce stress and support overall health. Chronic stress can hinder the body's detoxification processes, making stress reduction an essential aspect of natural detox techniques.

How to practice mindfulness and meditation:

- Find a quiet space and sit or lie down in a comfortable position.
- Focus your attention on your breath, a specific object, or a guided meditation.

- Let go of thoughts, worries, and stress as you become more present in the moment.

11. Fiber-Rich Foods

Fiber-rich foods are essential for promoting healthy digestion and supporting the elimination of waste products and toxins from the body. Soluble & insoluble fiber can help keep the digestive system functioning optimally.

Foods high in fiber:

- **Whole grains:** Oats, brown rice, quinoa, and whole wheat.
- **Legumes:** Beans, lentils, and chickpeas.
- **Fruits and vegetables:** Berries, apples, pears, leafy greens, and broccoli.

12. Lemon Water

Lemon water is a simple and natural detox technique that can support digestion and liver function. While lemon is acidic, it has an alkalizing effect on the body when metabolized, making it beneficial for maintaining a balanced pH.

How to make lemon water:

- Squeeze the juice of half a lemon into a glass of warm water.
- Drink this in the morning before eating to kickstart your digestive system.

13. Herbal Supplements

Certain herbal supplements can aid in detoxification. Herbs like milk thistle, dandelion root, and burdock root are believed to support liver function and overall detoxification processes.

Use herbal supplements with caution:

- If you choose to use herbal supplements, ensure they are of high quality and are taken under the guidance of a healthcare professional.
- Stay mindful of potential interactions with medications or pre-existing health conditions.

Dr. Sebi's Detox Plan

Dr. Sebi gained recognition for his unique dietary philosophy and herbal remedies, which he believed could detoxify the body, restore balance, and promote optimal health.

The Core Principles of Dr. Sebi's Detox Plan
Dr. Sebi's detox plan is grounded in several core principles that focus on nourishing the body with alkaline, natural, and unprocessed foods while eliminating acidic and harmful substances. These principles aim to support the body's innate detoxification processes and promote overall well-being. Here are the key principles of Dr. Sebi's detox plan:

1. **Alkaline Diet:** Dr. Sebi's detox plan centers around the consumption of alkaline-forming foods and beverages. He believed that maintaining a slightly alkaline pH in the body (around 7.35 to 7.45) is crucial for health and that acidic foods disrupt this balance. An alkaline diet focuses on fresh fruits, vegetables, nuts, seeds, and whole grains to create an alkaline environment in the body.

2. **Plant-Based Nutrition:** Dr. Sebi advocated for a plant-based diet, emphasizing the consumption of natural, unprocessed, and organic plant foods. He believed that plant-based foods were easier for the body to digest and assimilate, making them essential for overall health and detoxification.

3. **Elimination of Processed and Hybrid Foods:** Dr. Sebi's detox plan calls for the complete elimination of processed and hybrid foods from one's diet. He argued that these foods contain harmful additives and modifications that disrupt the body's natural healing processes. The focus is on consuming non-hybrid, non-GMO, and organic foods.

4. **Raw and Uncooked Foods:** Dr. Sebi recommended the consumption of raw and uncooked foods to preserve their natural vitality and essential nutrients. He believed that cooking food at high temperatures destroyed these nutrients, making raw foods more beneficial for the body.

5. **Herbal Supplements:** In addition to dietary recommendations, Dr. Sebi's detox plan includes the use of herbal supplements and botanical remedies. He believed that specific herbs and plants possessed powerful healing properties that could detoxify the body, enhance the immune system, and restore balance to various bodily systems.

6. **Detoxification and Cellular Health:** Detoxification is a central theme in Dr. Sebi's approach. He emphasized the importance of consuming foods with natural detoxifying properties, like leafy greens, cruciferous vegetables, and specific herbs and spices known for their cleansing and purifying effects.

7. **Hydration and Alkaline Water:** Proper hydration is vital in Dr. Sebi's detox plan. He recommended the consumption of alkaline water to balance the body's pH levels and support overall health. Alkaline water is thought to have a higher pH level than regular water, making it more alkaline and beneficial for the body.

Dr. Sebi's detox plan places a strong emphasis on specific dietary recommendations, with a focus on alkaline foods and the elimination of acidic and harmful substances. Here are some key dietary recommendations associated with his detox plan:

Alkaline Foods

- Fruits: Consume a variety of fresh fruits, including berries, apples, pears, and citrus fruits. These fruits are alkaline-forming and rich in essential nutrients.
- Vegetables: Fill your plate with colorful vegetables, like leafy greens, broccoli, carrots, bell peppers, and squash.
- Nuts and Seeds: Incorporate almonds, walnuts, chia seeds, and flaxseeds into your meals and snacks.
- Legumes: Include beans, lentils, and chickpeas to your diet for plant-based protein.
- Whole Grains: Choose whole grains like quinoa, brown rice, and oats for a healthier source of carbohydrates.

Elimination of Acidic Foods

- Animal Products: Dr. Sebi recommended reducing or eliminating meat, dairy, and eggs from your diet. Consider plant-based alternatives if transitioning to a vegan or vegetarian diet.
- Processed Foods: Limit or eliminate processed and highly refined foods, including sugary snacks, fast food, and packaged convenience meals.
- Sugar and Caffeine: Reduce your intake of sugary foods and beverages, and consider replacing coffee with herbal tea or alkaline water.

Raw and Uncooked Foods

- Dr. Sebi encouraged the consumption of raw fruits and vegetables, nuts, seeds, and grains to maximize the intake of essential nutrients and enzymes necessary for promoting optimal health.

Herbal Supplements in Dr. Sebi's Detox Plan
Dr. Sebi formulated and recommended his own line of herbal supplements to complement his dietary recommendations and support the body's natural detoxification processes. These herbal supplements were designed to address specific health concerns and promote overall well-being. Here are some of the herbal supplements commonly associated with Dr. Sebi's detox plan:

1. **Viento:** Viento is a herbal supplement that Dr. Sebi recommended to support respiratory health and improve overall well-being.

2. **Bio Ferro:** Bio Ferro is formulated to enhance the immune system, detoxify the blood, and promote healthy cellular function.

3. **Uterine Wash and Prostate Formula:** Dr. Sebi's detox plan included herbal supplements specifically designed for women's and men's health. The Uterine Wash and Prostate Formula were recommended to address gender-specific health concerns.

4. **Green Food Plus:** Green Food Plus is a nutritional supplement aimed at providing essential vitamins, minerals, and nutrients to support overall health and vitality.

5. **Sea Moss/Irish Moss:** Sea moss, also known as Irish moss, was promoted by Dr. Sebi for its nutrient-rich properties and its ability to support digestion and overall health.

6. **Nopal:** Nopal, a type of prickly pear cactus, is included in Dr. Sebi's detox plan for its potential to aid digestion, control blood sugar levels, and support detoxification.

7. **Bromide Plus:** Bromide Plus is recommended for its potential to support thyroid health, boost the immune system, and provide essential nutrients.

Important Considerations for Dr. Sebi's Detox Plan
While Dr. Sebi's detox plan has gained popularity among some individuals seeking alternative approaches to health and well-being, it is essential to approach it with a balanced perspective. Here are some essential considerations:

1. **Individual Variation:** Because each person is unique, strategies that work well for one person might not be appropriate for others. It's crucial to consider your own health status, dietary preferences, and any underlying medical conditions before adopting any detox plan, including Dr. Sebi's approach.

2. **Lack of Scientific Evidence:** Dr. Sebi's dietary and herbal recommendations are not supported by robust scientific evidence. While many people have reported positive experiences, the lack of scientific validation should be taken into account when considering this plan.

3. **Consultation with a Healthcare Professional:** Prior to making significant modifications to your diet or incorporating herbal supplements, it is prudent to consult with a your healthcare professional or a registered dietitian. They can offer personalized recommendations and ensure that your dietary decisions are in harmony with your health objectives.

4. **Gradual Transition:** Transitioning to an alkaline and plant-based diet should be done gradually. Sudden dietary changes can

lead to digestive disturbances, so it's advisable to take your time when adopting Dr. Sebi's recommendations.

Chapter 4:

The Detoxification Voyage

In this chapter, we will delve into the intricacies of detoxification, understanding its significance within the context of the alkaline diet. Prepare to embrace a 28-day detox plan, equipped with strategies to handle potential side effects and maximize the benefits of this rejuvenating process. Let us navigate through the stages of this detoxification voyage.

Week 1: Introduction to Alkaline Foods

In Week 1, we embark on our detoxification journey by acquainting ourselves with alkaline foods, the core of Dr. Sebi's detox plan. These foods lay the foundation for restoring health and well-being by balancing your body's pH levels and creating an environment unfavorable for diseases.

Day 1: Preparing for Your Detox

Your detox journey begins with a focus on preparation. Start your day with a simple yet powerful ritual: a glass of warm water with a squeeze of lemon. This combination helps kickstart your metabolism and primes your digestive system for the upcoming changes.

Herbal teas, like chamomile or ginger, can provide comfort to your digestive system. They are soothing, promote relaxation, and are caffeine-free, making them ideal for the morning.

Planning plays a pivotal role in achieving success in any detox program. On the first day, establish a positive foundation by preparing your meals for the week and crafting a grocery list. Make sure to prioritize alkaline foods like leafy greens, avocados, cucumbers, and other Dr. Sebi-approved items.

Day 2: The Alkaline Plate

Now that you've made a grocery list of alkaline foods, it's time to put them into action. Familiarize yourself with Dr. Sebi's recommended alkaline foods, like kale, spinach, and bell peppers. Aim to make these foods the star of your meals, constituting at least 80% of your plate.

By embracing these foods, you provide your body with an abundance of essential nutrients, minerals, and antioxidants, setting the stage for an effective detox.

Day 3: Eliminating Acidic Foods

In Day 3, we take a significant step toward detoxification by eliminating acidic foods from our diet. Acidic foods, like dairy, processed meats, and fried foods, can contribute to the accumulation of toxins in the body. Replace these items with healthier, alkaline alternatives, like almond milk and plant-based protein sources.

Eliminating acidic foods may challenge your taste buds initially, but it's a crucial step in creating an environment that supports your health & well-being.

Day 4: Hydration Matters

Proper hydration is essential throughout your detox journey. Today's focus is on staying hydrated with alkaline water and herbal teas. These beverages help flush toxins from your system and maintain the right pH balance in your body.

On the flip side, avoid sugary beverages and caffeinated drinks. These can introduce acidity and hinder the detoxification process.

Day 5: Detox Smoothies

A delightful way to integrate alkaline foods into your daily routine is by starting your day with a detoxifying smoothie. These nutrient-packed breakfasts can include components like kale, banana, and spirulina. Experiment with different combinations to find your favorites and kickstart your day with a burst of energy and vitality.

Day 6: Herbal Support

Herbs are nature's allies in detoxification. Day 6 introduces herbs like dandelion and burdock root into your diet. These herbs support the healthy functioning of your liver and kidneys, vital organs in the detox process. Relish these herbs as herbal teas throughout the day to harness their cleansing and healing properties.

Day 7: Rest and Reflect

After a week of gradual changes and mindful dietary shifts, it's time for a well-defined rest. On Day 7, take the opportunity to pause and reflect on your initial experiences with the detox plan.

Evaluate your energy levels, mood, and any noticeable changes in your body. These reflections can help motivate and guide you through the subsequent weeks of your detox journey.

Week 2: Deep Cleansing

Week 2 is where your body delves deeper into the detoxification process. This week is about cleansing, removing accumulated toxins and impurities, and preparing your body for the nourishment ahead.

Day 8: Introducing Fasting

Fasting is a time-honored practice that allows your digestive system to rest and intensify the detox process. On Day 8, consider a one-day fast consisting only of herbal teas and alkaline water. This fasting period can be an essential milestone in your detox journey.

Fasting can challenge your discipline but offers profound benefits. It gives your body an opportunity to eliminate stored toxins and reset its natural balance.

Day 9: The Power of Green Juices

Green juices are nutritional powerhouses that can significantly aid your detox. Incorporate them into your daily routine, using components like spinach, cucumber, and a touch of lime. These juices provide essential nutrients, vitamins, and antioxidants, contributing to the elimination of toxins and the rejuvenation of your body.

Day 10: Alkaline Grains

Day 10 introduces alkaline grains like quinoa, millet, and amaranth. These grains can replace acidic grains in your diet. Prepare them with alkaline herbs and seasonings to create flavorful, nutrient-rich dishes. These grains provide a steady source of energy while supporting the detox process.

Day 11: Healing Spices

Embrace the healing power of spices like turmeric and ginger on Day 11. These spices are well-known for their anti-inflammatory properties and can enhance the detoxification process. You can incorporate them into your cooking or steep them in teas for their beneficial effects.

Day 12: Colon Cleansing

The health of your colon is integral to the detox process. On Day 12, include psyllium husk or aloe vera in your daily regimen to support colon cleansing. However, it's crucial to maintain adequate hydration while using these remedies to ensure their effectiveness and avoid any discomfort.

Day 13: Sea Vegetables

Sea vegetables like dulse and nori are fantastic additions to your diet. These nutrient-dense marine plants are rich in minerals and can be used in various dishes, like soups, salads, or even as wraps. Their unique flavors and textures include a delightful twist to your meals while contributing to the detox process.

Day 14: Evaluate and Adjust

As you conclude Week 2, take a moment to evaluate and adjust. Reflect on the changes you've experienced during this deeper phase of detoxification. Notice any improvements in your energy levels, digestion, and overall well-being.

This reflection will help you understand the progress you've made and keep you motivated for the weeks ahead. Remember that detoxification is a journey, and each day takes you closer to your health goals.

Week 3: Nourishing Your Body

In Week 3, your body continues to detoxify while being nourished with a wide range of nutrient-rich foods. This week is all about nourishing and rejuvenating your body, ensuring it receives the vital nutrients necessary for optimal well-being.

Day 15: Protein Alternatives

On Day 15, you'll explore alternatives to animal protein. Plant-based sources like lentils, chickpeas, and tofu are rich in essential amino acids, which are vital for maintaining and repairing tissues. These alternatives provide a sustainable source of protein while aligning with the alkaline principles of the detox plan.

Day 16: Fresh Fruit Feast

Day 16 is a day to celebrate the vibrant flavors and nutrition of fresh fruits. Dedicate this day to consuming an array of alkaline fruits like papayas, berries, and watermelon. These fruits provide a plethora of vitamins, minerals, and antioxidants to support your health and rejuvenation.

Day 17: Detoxifying Teas

Your detox journey continues with detoxifying teas on Day 17. Continue to relish herbal teas like sarsaparilla and valerian root, which promote the elimination of toxins and support your overall well-being. These teas offer a soothing and therapeutic experience, making them an essential part of your detox routine.

Day 18: Nutrient-Packed Salads

Salads are a fantastic way to incorporate an array of alkaline foods into your diet. On Day 18, create a hearty alkaline salad using a variety of greens, vegetables, and herbs. Drizzle with olive oil & lemon juice for a zesty dressing that enhances the flavors and nutritional value of your meal.

Day 19: Alkaline Snacks

In Day 19, shift your focus to snacking. Replace processed and unhealthy snacks with more nourishing alternatives like almonds, pumpkin seeds, and dried fruits. These snacks offer sustained energy and satiety while aligning with the alkaline principles of your detox plan.

Day 20: Alkaline Soups

Alkaline soups are a delightful way to nourish your body. Explore alkaline soup recipes on Day 20, using components like okra, kale, and onions. Homemade vegetable broths include depth of flavor to your soups while providing essential nutrients. These soups are both comforting and beneficial for your detox journey.

Day 21: Reflection and Renewal

As you approach the end of Week 3, take some time for reflection and renewal. Reflect on your journey so far, the progress you've made, and how you feel physically and mentally. This reflection is essential for renewing your commitment to the detox plan for the final week, where you'll establish this transformative lifestyle.

Remember that your body has been through a significant detoxification process, and the nourishment you've provided it during this week has laid a strong foundation for your long-term well-being.

Week 4: Establishing the Lifestyle

In the final week, you'll solidify the detox plan as a long-term lifestyle change. This week is about building habits and practices that will support your health and well-being in the future.

Day 22: Intermittent Fasting

Intermittent fasting is a practice that many find beneficial for overall health. On Day 22, incorporate intermittent fasting into your daily routine. This approach allows your digestive system to rest during specific time windows and can promote detoxification. Choose a fasting window that aligns with your schedule and preferences.

Day 23: Alkaline Lifestyle Habits

Your lifestyle plays a significant role in your overall well-being. On Day 23, focus on implementing alkaline lifestyle habits. This includes stress reduction techniques like meditation, deep breathing exercises, and creating a calming bedtime routine for better sleep quality. These practices promote relaxation and support your body's natural detox processes.

Day 24: Alkaline Cooking Techniques

On Day 24, delve into alkaline cooking techniques. These methods, like steaming, baking, and grilling, retain the nutrient content of your food while maintaining alkalinity. Incorporating these techniques into your cooking ensures that you continue to prepare delicious and nutritious meals that align with your detox plan.

Day 25: Herbal Supplements

Consider incorporating herbal supplements into your diet on Day 25. However, it's crucial to do this under the guidance of a healthcare professional or knowledgeable herbalist. Herbal supplements can enhance the detoxification process, but their use should be tailored to your individual needs and goals.

Day 26: Alkaline Hydration

Proper hydration remains a top priority on Day 26. Continue to prioritize alkaline water and herbal teas, avoiding bottled water with low pH levels. Alkaline hydration ensures that your body maintains the right pH balance and supports detoxification.

Day 27: Celebrate Progress

On Day 27, take a moment to celebrate the progress you've made during your detox journey. Recognize the positive changes in your energy levels, skin, digestion, and overall well-being. Your commitment to better health is yielding results, and it's essential to acknowledge and appreciate your efforts.

Day 28: Long-Term Commitment

In your final day of the 28-day detox plan, make a commitment to a long-term alkaline lifestyle. This commitment involves prioritizing alkaline foods, herbs, and holistic health practices in your daily life. Your journey to better health is not confined to 28 days but is a lifelong endeavor that you are now well-equipped to embrace.

Handling Potential Side Effects

Throughout your 28-day detox journey, you may encounter side effects like headaches, fatigue, or digestive discomfort. Here are strategies to manage them:

1. **Stay Hydrated:** Proper hydration is a fundamental strategy to alleviate many detox-related symptoms. Continue to drink alkaline water and herbal teas consistently to help your body eliminate toxins.

2. **Gradual Transition:** If you find the detox process challenging, consider a gradual transition into Dr. Sebi's diet to minimize discomfort. Give your body time to adjust to the changes.

3. **Consult a Professional:** If you have underlying health conditions or are unsure about specific aspects of the detox plan, consult a healthcare professional or a nutritionist. They can provide personalized guidance and support.

4. **Monitor Your Body:** Pay close attention to your body's signals. If you experience severe discomfort or unusual symptoms, it's essential to be responsive and adapt your detox plan as needed.

5. **Supportive Community:** Consider joining a supportive community or engaging with like-minded individuals who are also on a detox journey. Sharing experiences, tips, and motivation can be invaluable in staying on track and achieving your health goals.

Chapter 5:

Sip the Nectar of Nature

Welcome to a world where health and taste harmoniously intertwine. In this chapter, we unveil a treasure trove of juice and smoothie recipes that transcend the boundaries of mere sustenance, transforming into potent potions of health and a celebration of taste and wellness. Prepare to immerse yourself in a collection of 50 Alkaline & Anti-Inflammatory Smoothie and Juice Recipes that will tantalize your taste buds and nourish your body.

50 Alkaline & Anti-Inflammatory Smoothie and Juice Recipes

1. *Green Goddess Detox Smoothie*
Preparation time: 5 mins

Servings: 2

Ingredients:

- 2 teacups fresh spinach leaves
- 1 ripe banana
- 1/2 cucumber
- 1/2 lemon (juiced)
- 1 teacup coconut water
- 1 tbsp chia seeds (elective)

Directions:

1. Include the entire components to a mixer.

2. Blend till smooth.

3. Pour into glasses and present instantly.

Per serving: Calories: 120kcal; Carbs: 26g; Protein: 3g; Sugar: 10g

2. *Blueberry Bliss Antioxidant Juice*
Preparation time: 10 mins

Servings: 2

Ingredients:

- 2 teacups blueberries (fresh or frozen)
- 1/2 teacup kale leaves
- 1/2 lemon (juiced)
- 1 teacup water

Directions:

1. Blend the entire components inside a mixer.

2. Blend till smooth.

3. Strain the mixture to take out any pulp.

4. Pour into glasses and present chilled.

Per serving: Calories: 60kcal; Carbs: 15g; Protein: 1g; Sugar: 9g

3. *Pineapple Paradise Anti-Inflammatory Shake*
Preparation time: 5 mins

Servings: 1

Ingredients:

- 1 teacup pineapple chunks
- 1/2 banana
- 1/2 teacup coconut milk
- 1/2 tsp ground ginger
- 1 tbsp agave syrup (elective)

Directions:

1. Blend the entire components inside a mixer.

2. Blend till smooth.

3. Include agave syrup for sweetness if anticipated.

4. Present in a glass.

Per serving: Calories: 250kcal; Carbs: 54g; Protein: 3g; Sugar: 35g

4. Alkaline Apple Cider Vinegar Drink
Preparation time: 2 mins

Servings: 1

Ingredients:

- 1 tbsp apple cider vinegar
- 1 teacup water
- 1 tbsp lemon juice
- 1 tsp agave syrup (elective)

Directions:

1. Mix apple cider vinegar, water, and lemon juice in a glass.

2. Include agave syrup for sweetness if anticipated.

3. Stir well and present.

Per serving: Calories: 15kcal; Carbs: 4g; Protein: 0g; Sugar: 3g

5. *Immunity Boosting Berry Blast*
Preparation time: 5 mins

Servings: 2

Ingredients:

- 1 teacup mixed berries (strawberries, blueberries, raspberries)
- 1 banana
- 1/2 teacup almond yogurt
- 1 tbsp agave syrup
- 1/2 teacup water or almond milk

Directions:

1. Blend the entire components inside a mixer.

2. Blend till smooth.

3. Pour into glasses and relish.

Per serving: Calories: 180kcal; Carbs: 40g; Protein: 5g; Sugar: 26g

6. *Kale and Kiwi Alkalizing Smoothie*
Preparation time: 5 mins

Servings: 1

Ingredients:

- 1 teacup severed kale leaves
- 2 ripe kiwis, skinned and carved
- 1/2 banana
- 1 teacup coconut water
- 1 tbsp chia seeds (elective)

Directions:

1. Put the entire components inside a mixer.

2. Blend till smooth.

3. Present instantly.

Per serving: Calories: 220kcal; Carbs: 49g; Protein: 6g; Sugar: 27g

7. Ginger Zest Anti-Inflammatory Elixir
Preparation time: 5 mins

Servings: 1

Ingredients:

- 1 teacup water
- 1-inch piece of fresh ginger, grated
- 1 tbsp lemon juice
- 1 tsp agave syrup

Directions:

1. Warm the water and ginger inside a small saucepot till it simmers.

2. Take out from heat then place lemon juice and agave syrup.

3. Stir well and present hot.

Per serving: Calories: 25kcal; Carbs: 6g; Protein: 0g; Sugar: 4g

8. Mango Magic Anti-Inflammatory Smoothie
Preparation time: 5 mins

Servings: 2

Ingredients:

- 2 ripe mangoes, skinned and cubed
- 1/2 teacup plain almond yogurt
- 1/2 teacup coconut milk
- 1 tbsp agave syrup (elective)

Directions:

1. Blend the entire components inside a mixer.

2. Blend till smooth.

3. Include agave syrup for extra sweetness if anticipated.

4. Pour into glasses and present.

Per serving: Calories: 220kcal; Carbs: 43g; Protein: 7g; Sugar: 36g

9. *Cucumber Cool Down Juice*
Preparation time: 5 mins

Servings: 1

Ingredients:

- 1 cucumber
- 1/2 lemon (juiced)
- 1/2 tsp fresh mint leaves
- 1 teacup water

Directions:

1. Slice the cucumber and put it inside a mixer.

2. Include lemon juice, mint leaves, and water.

3. Blend till smooth.

4. Present chilled.

Per serving: Calories: 15kcal; Carbs: 4g; Protein: 0g; Sugar: 2g

10. Citrus Sunshine Detox Shake
Preparation time: 5 mins

Servings: 1

Ingredients:

- 1 orange, skinned and segmented
- 1/2 grapefruit, skinned and segmented
- 1/2 lemon (juiced)
- 1/2 lime (juiced)
- 1/2 teacup coconut water
- 1 tbsp agave syrup (elective)

Directions:

1. Blend the entire components inside a mixer.

2. Blend till smooth.

3. Include agave syrup for sweetness if anticipated.

4. Pour into a glass and relish.

Per serving: Calories: 120kcal; Carbs: 30g; Protein: 2g; Sugar: 20g

11. Berry Beet Bliss Smoothie
Preparation time: 5 mins

Servings: 2

Ingredients:

- 1 teacup mixed berries (strawberries, blueberries, raspberries)
- 1 small beet, skinned and cubed
- 1 banana

- 1 teacup almond milk
- 1 tbsp agave syrup (elective)

Directions:

1. Blend the entire components inside a mixer.

2. Blend till smooth.

3. Sweeten with agave syrup if anticipated.

4. Pour into glasses and present.

Per serving: Calories: 150kcal; Carbs: 36g; Protein: 3g; Sugar: 22g

12. Carrot Turmeric Tonic
Preparation time: 5 mins

Servings: 1

Ingredients:

- 2 medium carrots, severed
- 1/2 tsp ground turmeric
- 1/2 inch fresh ginger, grated
- 1/2 lemon (juiced)
- 1 teacup water

Directions:

1. Blend carrots, turmeric, ginger, and water inside a mixer.

2. Blend till smooth.

3. Include lemon juice and blend thoroughly.

4. Present chilled or over ice.

Per serving: Calories: 70kcal; Carbs: 17g; Protein: 2g; Sugar: 8g

13. Spinach and Pineapple Green Smoothie
Preparation time: 5 mins

Servings: 1

Ingredients:

- 1 teacup fresh spinach leaves
- 1 teacup pineapple chunks
- 1/2 banana
- 1/2 teacup coconut water
- 1 tbsp chia seeds (elective)

Directions:

1. Put the entire components inside a mixer.

2. Blend till smooth.

3. Include chia seeds for extra texture and nutrition, if anticipated.

4. Present instantly.

Per serving: Calories: 190kcal; Carbs: 45g; Protein: 3g; Sugar: 29g

14. Lemon Ginger Immune Booster
Preparation time: 5 mins

Servings: 1

Ingredients:

- 1 teacup water
- 1/2 lemon (juiced)
- 1/2 inch fresh ginger, grated
- 1 tsp agave syrup (elective)

Directions:

1. Mix water, lemon juice, and grated ginger in a glass.

2. Sweeten with agave syrup if anticipated.

3. Stir well and present.

Per serving: Calories: 20kcal; Carbs: 6g; Protein: 0g; Sugar: 4g

15. Watermelon Wonder Juice
Preparation time: 5 mins

Servings: 2

Ingredients:

- 4 teacups fresh watermelon, cubed
- 1/2 lime (juiced)
- 1/4 teacup fresh mint leaves
- Ice cubes (elective)

Directions:

1. Put the watermelon, lime juice, and fresh mint inside a mixer.

2. Blend till smooth.

3. Include ice cubes for a chilled version.

4. Pour into glasses then garnish with extra mint leaves.

Per serving: Calories: 80kcal; Carbs: 20g; Protein: 1g; Sugar: 17g

16. Avocado Alkaline Elixir
Preparation time: 5 mins

Servings: 1

Ingredients:

- 1 ripe avocado
- 1 teacup spinach leaves
- 1/2 cucumber
- 1/2 lemon (juiced)
- 1 teacup water

Directions:

1. Blend the avocado, spinach, cucumber, lemon juice, and water inside a mixer.

2. Blend till smooth.

3. Pour into a glass and present.

Per serving: Calories: 250kcal; Carbs: 18g; Protein: 4g; Sugar: 3g

17. Sweet Potato Spice Smoothie
Preparation time: 5 mins

Servings: 2

Ingredients:

- 2 teacups cooked and cooled sweet potato, mashed
- 1 teacup almond milk
- 1/2 tsp ground cinnamon
- 1/4 tsp ground nutmeg
- 1 tbsp maple syrup (elective)

Directions:

1. Blend the sweet potato, almond milk, cinnamon, and nutmeg inside a mixer.

2. Blend till smooth.

3. Sweeten with maple syrup, if anticipated.

4. Pour into glasses and relish.

Per serving: Calories: 150kcal; Carbs: 36g; Protein: 2g; Sugar: 9g

18. *Cherry Almond Delight*
Preparation time: 5 mins

Servings: 1

Ingredients:

- 1 teacup frozen cherries
- 1/2 teacup almond milk
- 1/4 teacup plain almond yogurt
- 1 tbsp almond butter
- 1 tsp agave syrup (elective)

Directions:

1. Blend frozen cherries, almond milk, almond yogurt, almond butter, and agave syrup inside a mixer.

2. Blend till smooth.

3. Sweeten with agave syrup if anticipated.

4. Present in a glass.

Per serving: Calories: 250kcal; Carbs: 28g; Protein: 9g; Sugar: 17g

19. *Aloe Vera Euphoria Juice*
Preparation time: 5 mins

Servings: 1

Ingredients:

- 1/4 teacup fresh aloe vera gel
- 1/2 cucumber
- 1/2 lemon (juiced)
- 1 teacup water
- 1 tsp agave syrup (elective)

Directions:

1. Place aloe vera gel, cucumber, lemon juice, water, and agave syrup inside a mixer.

2. Blend till smooth.

3. Sweeten with agave syrup, if anticipated.

4. Present chilled.

Per serving: Calories: 25kcal; Carbs: 7g; Protein: 1g; Sugar: 3g

20. Pear Perfection Anti-Inflammatory Shake
Preparation time: 5 mins

Servings: 1

Ingredients:

- 1 ripe pear, skinned and eroded
- 1/2 teacup unsweetened almond milk
- 1/2 tsp ground cinnamon
- 1/2 tsp agave syrup (elective)

Directions:

1. Slice the pear and put it inside a mixer.

2. Include almond milk, ground cinnamon, and agave syrup (if anticipated).

3. Blend till smooth.

4. Pour into a glass and present.

Per serving: Calories: 100kcal; Carbs: 26g; Protein: 1g; Sugar: 17g

21. Red Cabbage Cleansing Smoothie
Preparation time: 5 mins

Servings: 2

Ingredients:

- 1 teacup severed red cabbage
- 1 apple, eroded and severed
- 1/2 lemon (juiced)
- 1 teacup water
- 1 tbsp agave syrup (elective)

Directions:

1. Blend red cabbage, apple, lemon juice, and water inside a mixer.

2. Blend till smooth.

3. Sweeten with agave syrup if anticipated.

4. Pour into glasses and relish.

Per serving: Calories: 70kcal; Carbs: 18g; Protein: 1g; Sugar: 12g

22. Golden Milk Turmeric Smoothie
Preparation time: 5 mins

Servings: 1

Ingredients:

- 1 teacup unsweetened coconut milk

- 1/2 tsp ground turmeric
- 1/2 tsp ground cinnamon
- 1/4 tsp ground black pepper
- 1 banana
- 1 tsp agave syrup (elective)

Directions:

1. Blend coconut milk, turmeric, cinnamon, black pepper, banana, and agave syrup inside a mixer.

2. Blend till smooth.

3. Include agave syrup for sweetness if anticipated.

4. Present in a glass.

Per serving: Calories: 180kcal; Carbs: 38g; Protein: 2g; Sugar: 19g

23. Cranberry Cleanse Juice
Preparation time: 10 mins

Servings: 2

Ingredients:

- 1 teacup fresh cranberries
- 1 apple, eroded and severed
- 1/2 orange (juiced)
- 1 teacup water
- 1 tbsp agave syrup (elective)

Directions:

1. Place cranberries, apple, orange juice, and water inside a mixer.

2. Blend till smooth.

3. Sweeten with agave syrup if anticipated.

4. Pour into glasses and present chilled.

Per serving: Calories: 70kcal; Carbs: 19g; Protein: 1g; Sugar: 13g

24. Kiwi Kale Kickstart
Preparation time: 5 mins

Servings: 1

Ingredients:

- 2 kiwis, skinned and carved
- 1 teacup severed kale leaves
- 1/2 banana
- 1/2 teacup water

Directions:

1. Blend kiwis, kale, banana, and water inside a mixer.

2. Blend till smooth.

3. Pour into a glass and present.

Per serving: Calories: 150kcal; Carbs: 37g; Protein: 4g; Sugar: 19g

25. Almond Blueberry Bliss Shake
Preparation time: 5 mins

Servings: 1

Ingredients:

- 1 teacup almond milk
- 1/2 teacup fresh or frozen blueberries
- 1 ripe banana

- 1 tbsp almond butter
- 1/2 tsp agave syrup (elective)

Directions:

1. Blend almond milk, blueberries, banana, almond butter, and agave syrup (if anticipated) inside a mixer.

2. Blend till smooth.

3. Pour into a glass and present.

Per serving: Calories: 280kcal; Carbs: 45g; Protein: 4g; Sugar: 27g

26. Carrot-Ginger Elixir
Preparation time: 5 mins

Servings: 1

Ingredients:

- 2 medium carrots, severed
- 1-inch piece of fresh ginger, grated
- 1/2 lemon (juiced)
- 1 teacup water

Directions:

1. Blend carrots, ginger, lemon juice, and water inside a mixer.

2. Blend till smooth.

3. Present chilled or over ice.

Per serving: Calories: 50kcal; Carbs: 12g; Protein: 1g; Sugar: 4g

27. Papaya Passion Anti-Inflammatory Smoothie
Preparation time: 5 mins

Servings: 2

Ingredients:

- 1 teacup fresh papaya chunks
- 1/2 teacup pineapple chunks
- 1/2 tsp ground turmeric
- 1/2 teacup coconut milk
- 1 tbsp agave syrup (elective)

Directions:

1. Place papaya, pineapple, turmeric, coconut milk, and agave syrup (if anticipated) inside a mixer.

2. Blend till smooth.

3. Pour into glasses and relish.

Per serving: Calories: 150kcal; Carbs: 36g; Protein: 1g; Sugar: 29g

28. Minty Melon Refresher
Preparation time: 5 mins

Servings: 1

Ingredients:

- 1 teacup fresh melon (e.g., cantaloupe or honeydew), cubed
- 1/2 teacup fresh mint leaves
- 1/2 lime (juiced)
- 1 teacup water
- 1 tsp agave syrup (elective)

Directions:

1. Blend melon, mint leaves, lime juice, water, and agave syrup inside a mixer.

2. Blend till smooth.

3. Sweeten with agave syrup if anticipated.

4. Present chilled.

Per serving: Calories: 60kcal; Carbs: 15g; Protein: 1g; Sugar: 11g

29. *Red Pepper Rejuvenation Juice*
Preparation time: 5 mins

Servings: 1

Ingredients:

- 1 red bell pepper, seeds taken out & severed
- 1/2 lemon (juiced)
- 1/2 cucumber
- 1 teacup water

Directions:

1. Place red bell pepper, lemon juice, cucumber, and water inside a mixer.

2. Blend till smooth.

3. Present instantly.

Per serving: Calories: 30kcal; Carbs: 7g; Protein: 1g; Sugar: 3g

30. *Pineapple Turmeric Tonic*
Preparation time: 5 mins

Servings: 1

Ingredients:

- 1 teacup fresh pineapple chunks
- 1/2 tsp ground turmeric
- 1/2 teacup coconut water
- 1/2 lemon (juiced)
- 1 tsp agave syrup (elective)

Directions:

1. Blend pineapple, turmeric, coconut water, lemon juice, and agave syrup inside a mixer.

2. Blend till smooth.

3. Sweeten with agave syrup if anticipated.

4. Present in a glass.

Per serving: Calories: 120kcal; Carbs: 30g; Protein: 2g; Sugar: 20g

31. Cilantro Detox Elixir
Preparation time: 5 mins

Servings: 1

Ingredients:

- 1 teacup fresh cilantro leaves
- 1/2 cucumber
- 1/2 lemon (juiced)
- 1/2 inch fresh ginger, grated
- 1 teacup water

Directions:

1. Blend cilantro, cucumber, lemon juice, ginger, and water inside a mixer.

2. Blend till smooth.

3. Present chilled or over ice.

Per serving: Calories: 20kcal; Carbs: 5g; Protein: 1g; Sugar: 2g

32. Raspberry Radiance Smoothie
Preparation time: 5 mins

Servings: 1

Ingredients:

- 1 teacup fresh raspberries
- 1/2 teacup plain almond yogurt
- 1/2 teacup almond milk
- 1 tbsp agave syrup
- 1/2 tsp vanilla extract

Directions:

1. Blend raspberries, almond yogurt, almond milk, agave syrup, and vanilla extract inside a mixer.

2. Blend till smooth.

3. Pour into a glass and present.

Per serving: Calories: 180kcal; Carbs: 32g; Protein: 10g; Sugar: 23g

33. Lemon Basil Alkaline Juice
Preparation time: 5 mins

Servings: 1

Ingredients:

- 2 lemons (juiced)
- Handful of fresh basil leaves
- 1 teacup water
- 1 tsp agave syrup (elective)

Directions:

1. Blend lemon juice, basil leaves, water, and agave syrup (if anticipated) inside a mixer.

2. Blend till smooth.

3. Pour into a glass and present.

Per serving: Calories: 30kcal; Carbs: 10g; Protein: 1g; Sugar: 5g

34. Orange Carrot Crush
Preparation time: 5 mins

Servings: 1

Ingredients:

- 2 large carrots, severed
- 2 oranges (juiced)
- 1/2 lemon (juiced)
- 1/2 inch fresh ginger, grated
- Ice cubes (elective)

Directions:

1. Blend severed carrots, orange juice, lemon juice, grated ginger, and ice cubes (if anticipated) inside a mixer.

2. Blend till smooth.

3. Pour into a glass and relish.

Per serving: Calories: 80kcal; Carbs: 20g; Protein: 2g; Sugar: 12g

35. *Mango Mint Magic*
Preparation time: 5 mins

Servings: 1

Ingredients:

- 1 ripe mango, skinned and cubed
- Handful of fresh mint leaves
- 1/2 teacup coconut milk
- 1/2 teacup water
- 1 tsp agave syrup (elective)

Directions:

1. Blend mango, mint leaves, coconut milk, water, and agave syrup (if anticipated) inside a mixer.

2. Blend till smooth.

3. Pour into a glass and present.

Per serving: Calories: 250kcal; Carbs: 54g; Protein: 3g; Sugar: 45g

36. *Blue Spirulina Bliss Smoothie*
Preparation time: 5 mins

Servings: 1

Ingredients:

- 1 ripe banana
- 1 teacup almond milk
- 1 tsp blue spirulina powder
- 1 tbsp agave syrup (elective)

Directions:

1. Blend the banana, almond milk, blue spirulina powder, and agave syrup (if anticipated) inside a mixer.

2. Blend till smooth.

3. Pour into a glass and present.

Per serving: Calories: 180kcal; Carbs: 43g; Protein: 2g; Sugar: 26g

37. Strawberry Fields Forever Juice
Preparation time: 5 mins

Servings: 1

Ingredients:

- 1 teacup fresh strawberries
- 1/2 teacup water
- 1/2 lemon (juiced)
- 1 tsp agave syrup (elective)

Directions:

1. Blend fresh strawberries, water, lemon juice, and agave syrup (if anticipated) inside a mixer.

2. Blend till smooth.

3. Pour into a glass and present.

Per serving: Calories: 60kcal; Carbs: 15g; Protein: 1g; Sugar: 9g

38. Peach Paradise Alkaline Smoothie
Preparation time: 5 mins

Servings: 1

Ingredients:

- 1 ripe peach, skinned and carved
- 1 teacup spinach leaves
- 1/2 teacup almond milk
- 1/2 banana
- 1 tsp agave syrup (elective)

Directions:

1. Blend the carved peach, spinach leaves, almond milk, banana, and agave syrup (if anticipated) inside a mixer.

2. Blend till smooth.

3. Pour into a glass and present.

Per serving: Calories: 160kcal; Carbs: 38g; Protein: 3g; Sugar: 25g

39. Beetroot Beauty Shake
Preparation time: 5 mins

Servings: 1

Ingredients:

- 1 small beetroot, skinned and cubed
- 1/2 teacup almond yogurt
- 1/2 teacup almond milk
- 1 tbsp agave syrup
- 1/2 tsp vanilla extract

Directions:

1. Blend cubed beetroot, almond yogurt, almond milk, agave syrup, and vanilla extract inside a mixer.

2. Blend till smooth.

3. Pour into a glass and relish.

Per serving: Calories: 220kcal; Carbs: 45g; Protein: 7g; Sugar: 35g

40. Matcha Green Tea Delight
Preparation time: 5 mins

Servings: 1

Ingredients:

- 1 tsp matcha green tea powder
- 1 teacup almond milk
- 1/2 banana
- 1 tsp agave syrup (elective)

Directions:

1. Blend matcha green tea powder, almond milk, banana, and agave syrup (if anticipated) inside a mixer.

2. Blend till smooth.

3. Pour into a glass and present.

Per serving: Calories: 150kcal; Carbs: 28g; Protein: 3g; Sugar: 19g

41. Cherry Chia Chiller
Preparation time: 5 mins

Servings: 1

Ingredients:

- 1 teacup fresh or frozen cherries
- 1 teacup coconut water

- 1 tbsp chia seeds
- 1/2 tsp agave syrup (elective)

Directions:

1. Blend cherries, coconut water, chia seeds, and agave syrup (if anticipated) inside a mixer.

2. Blend till smooth.

3. Pour into a glass and present.

Per serving: Calories: 150kcal; Carbs: 34g; Protein: 3g; Sugar: 22g

42. Green Apple Ginger Glow
Preparation time: 5 mins

Servings: 1

Ingredients:

- 1 green apple, eroded and carved
- 1/2 inch fresh ginger, grated
- 1 teacup water
- 1/2 lemon (juiced)
- 1 tsp agave syrup (elective)

Directions:

1. Blend green apple, grated ginger, water, lemon juice, and agave syrup inside a mixer.

2. Blend till smooth.

3. Pour into a glass and relish.

Per serving: Calories: 60kcal; Carbs: 16g; Protein: 1g; Sugar: 11g

43. Pineapple Parsley Power Juice
Preparation time: 5 mins

Servings: 1

Ingredients:

- 1 teacup fresh pineapple chunks
- Handful of fresh parsley leaves
- 1/2 lemon (juiced)
- 1/2 cucumber
- 1/2 tsp agave syrup (elective)

Directions:

1. Place pineapple chunks, parsley leaves, lemon juice, cucumber, and agave syrup inside a mixer.

2. Blend till smooth.

3. Pour into a glass and present chilled.

Per serving: Calories: 70kcal; Carbs: 19g; Protein: 2g; Sugar: 11g

44. Spinach Sunshine Elixir
Preparation time: 5 mins

Servings: 1

Ingredients:

- 1 teacup fresh spinach leaves
- 1 orange (juiced)
- 1/2 teacup water
- 1/2 tsp agave syrup (elective)

Directions:

1. Blend spinach leaves, orange juice, water, and agave syrup (if anticipated) inside a mixer.

2. Blend till smooth.

3. Pour into a glass and relish.

Per serving: Calories: 40kcal; Carbs: 10g; Protein: 2g; Sugar: 6g

45. *Apricot Alkaline Ambrosia*
Preparation time: 5 mins

Servings: 1

Ingredients:

- 1 teacup fresh apricots, pitted
- 1/2 banana
- 1/2 teacup coconut water
- 1 tsp agave syrup (elective)

Directions:

1. Blend apricots, banana, coconut water, and agave syrup inside a mixer.

2. Blend till smooth.

3. Pour into a glass and present.

Per serving: Calories: 160kcal; Carbs: 38g; Protein: 2g; Sugar: 25g

46. *Turmeric Pineapple Passion*
Preparation time: 5 mins

Servings: 1

Ingredients:

- 1 teacup fresh pineapple chunks
- 1/2 tsp ground turmeric
- 1/2 teacup coconut water
- 1/2 lemon (juiced)
- 1 tsp agave syrup (elective)

Directions:

1. Blend pineapple chunks, ground turmeric, coconut water, lemon juice, and agave syrup (if anticipated) inside a mixer.

2. Blend till smooth.

3. Pour into a glass and present.

Per serving: Calories: 80kcal; Carbs: 20g; Protein: 1g; Sugar: 13g

47. Acai Berry Antioxidant Smoothie
Preparation time: 5 mins

Servings: 1

Ingredients:

- 1 packet of frozen acai puree
- 1/2 teacup mixed berries (e.g., strawberries, blueberries, raspberries)
- 1 teacup almond milk
- 1 tbsp agave syrup
- 1/2 banana

Directions:

1. Blend the acai puree, mixed berries, almond milk, agave syrup, and banana inside a mixer.

2. Blend till smooth.

3. Pour into a glass and relish.

Per serving: Calories: 250kcal; Carbs: 55g; Protein: 3g; Sugar: 43g

48. Basil Berry Bliss Shake
Preparation time: 5 mins

Servings: 1

Ingredients:

- Handful of fresh basil leaves
- 1 teacup mixed berries (e.g., strawberries, blueberries, raspberries)
- 1 teacup almond milk
- 1 tsp agave syrup (elective)
- 1/2 banana

Directions:

1. Blend the basil leaves, mixed berries, almond milk, agave syrup, and banana inside a mixer.

2. Blend till smooth.

3. Pour into a glass and present.

Per serving: Calories: 200kcal; Carbs: 46g; Protein: 3g; Sugar: 29g

49. Lemon Lavender Serenity Elixir
Preparation time: 5 mins

Servings: 1

Ingredients:

- 1/2 lemon (juiced)
- 1/2 tsp dried lavender buds
- 1 teacup water

- 1 tsp agave syrup (elective)

Directions:

1. Blend lemon juice, dried lavender buds, water, and agave syrup (if anticipated) inside a mixer.

2. Blend till well mixed.

3. Pour into a glass and relish.

Per serving: Calories: 20kcal; Carbs: 6g; Protein: 1g; Sugar: 3g

50. Peach Turmeric Tango
Preparation time: 5 mins

Servings: 1

Ingredients:

- 1 ripe peach, skinned and carved
- 1/2 tsp ground turmeric
- 1/2 teacup coconut milk
- 1/2 teacup water
- 1 tsp agave syrup (elective)

Directions:

1. Blend the carved peach, ground turmeric, coconut milk, water, and agave syrup (if anticipated) inside a mixer.

2. Blend till smooth.

3. Pour into a glass and present.

Per serving: Calories: 140kcal; Carbs: 31g; Protein: 2g; Sugar: 22g

Chapter 6:

Transitioning to Tranquility

In this chapter, we equip you with insights and tips for smoothly transitioning from a standard diet to Dr. Sebi's alkaline diet, ensuring that you can overcome common hurdles and set the stage for a nourished life. Transitioning to a new way of eating can present challenges, but with the right knowledge and strategies, you can navigate this journey with ease. Let's explore how you can embrace tranquility through a seamless transition.

Transition Challenges and Overcoming Them

Transitioning from a standard diet to Dr. Sebi's alkaline diet can be a transformative journey for your health and well-being. While this dietary shift offers numerous benefits, it's not without its challenges.

1. Lack of Familiarity

One of the initial challenges when transitioning to Dr. Sebi's alkaline diet is the lack of familiarity with the foods and principles. Most people are accustomed to a diet that includes a significant amount of processed, acidic, and animal-based foods. Shifting to an entirely different way of eating can feel overwhelming.

How to Overcome:

- **Education:** Start by educating yourself about the alkaline diet. Learn about the principles, the importance of alkaline-forming foods, and why certain foods are discouraged.
- **Recipe Exploration:** Explore alkaline diet recipes to discover delicious and satisfying meals. There are plenty of resources, including cookbooks and websites, that offer creative recipes.
- **Gradual Transition:** Rather than making a sudden and complete switch, consider a gradual transition. Begin by incorporating more alkaline foods into your current diet and progressively reducing acidic ones.

2. **Cravings**

Cravings for familiar foods, especially those high in sugar, salt, and processed components, are common during the transition. Your taste buds are accustomed to certain flavors, and cravings can be strong.

How to Overcome:

- **Substitutes:** Find healthy substitutes for your cravings. For example, if you crave sweets, opt for fresh fruit. If you miss salty snacks, try roasted nuts or seaweed snacks.
- **Mindful Eating:** Practice mindful eating. Take the time to savor your food, paying attention to its flavors and textures. Mindful eating could aid in decreasing cravings.
- **Detox Support:** Consider herbal teas or supplements that can support your detox and help reduce cravings.

3. **Social Pressure**

Social gatherings, family events, and dining out with friends can be challenging when you're following a specific diet. You might face pressure from others to indulge in non-alkaline foods.

How to Overcome:

- **Communication:** Let your friends and family know about your dietary choices and the reasons behind them. Educating them about your commitment can reduce pressure.
- **Bring Your Own Dish:** If you're invited to a social event, offer to bring a dish that fits your diet. This ensures you have something to eat that aligns with your goals.
- **Research Dining Options:** When dining out, research restaurants that offer alkaline-friendly options. Many restaurants now cater to various dietary preferences.

4. **Nutritional Concerns**

As you transition to the alkaline diet, you may have concerns about meeting your nutritional needs, especially with the elimination of animal products.

How to Overcome:

- **Consult a Dietitian:** Consider consulting with a registered dietitian or nutritionist who is knowledgeable about plant-based diets. They can help you plan balanced meals and address any nutritional concerns.
- **Supplements:** If you're worried about specific nutrients, like vitamin B12, iron, or omega-3 fatty acids.
- **Diverse Diet:** Focus on a diverse and colorful diet. By incorporating a broad diversity of fruits, nuts, vegetables, and seeds, you can cover a broad spectrum of nutrients.

5. **Digestive Changes**

Shifting from a standard diet to an alkaline one can lead to digestive changes. You may experience more frequent bowel movements, bloating, or other digestive discomforts.

How to Overcome:

- **Hydration:** Ensure you're drinking plenty of water to stay hydrated, which is essential for healthy digestion.
- **Fiber Intake:** Slowly increase your fiber intake to let your digestive system to adapt to the change. Foods like chia seeds, flaxseeds, and leafy greens can be excellent sources of fiber.
- **Probiotics:** Consider adding probiotic-rich foods like sauerkraut or kimchi to your diet. Probiotics can help support digestive health.

6. **Emotional Changes**

The detoxification process can lead to emotional changes, including mood swings and irritability. This transition can be mentally challenging.

How to Overcome:

- **Mindfulness:** Engage in mindfulness practices like meditation, yoga, or deep breathing exercises to manage stress and emotional changes.
- **Support Network:** Connect with a support network of like-minded individuals who are also following the alkaline diet. Sharing your experiences & challenges with others can be therapeutic.
- **Patience:** Understand that emotional changes are part of the detoxification process. Be patient with yourself and acknowledge that these changes are temporary.

7. **Budget Constraints**

Another challenge you might encounter is budget constraints. Some people believe that eating healthily is expensive, but this isn't necessarily true.

How to Overcome:

- **Meal Planning:** Plan your meals in advance and create a budget-friendly shopping list. Meal planning can help you make cost-effective food choices.
- **Buy in Bulk:** Purchase non-perishable alkaline staples like rice, beans, and grains in bulk. This often reduces the cost per serving.
- **Local and Seasonal Foods:** Shop for locally grown and seasonal produce, which can be more affordable and fresher than imported options.

8. **Staying Committed**

Maintaining long-term commitment to Dr. Sebi's alkaline diet can be challenging, especially when faced with temptations and cravings.

How to Overcome:

- **Set Clear Goals:** Clearly define your reasons for adopting this diet. Having a strong sense of purpose can help you stay committed.
- **Track Your Progress:** Keep a journal to track your progress, including how you feel physically and emotionally. This can present as a motivator.
- **Seek Support:** Consider joining online communities or support groups dedicated to the alkaline diet. Sharing your journey and seeking support can boost your commitment.

Transitioning to Dr. Sebi's alkaline diet is a significant step toward improving your health and overall well-being. While there are challenges along the way, with the right strategies and support, you can overcome them and successfully make the shift to a lifestyle that promotes vitality and longevity. Remember that the journey is unique to each individual, and it is really necessary to pay attention to what your body is telling you and to make decisions that are in line with your individual requirements and inclinations.

What to Expect When Transitioning

Transitioning from a standard diet to Dr. Sebi's alkaline diet is a transformative journey that can lead to improved health and overall well-being. While the process can be rewarding, it's essential to understand what to expect during this transition. This section provides insights into the typical experiences and challenges individuals encounter when adopting Dr. Sebi's alkaline diet and offers practical advice on how to navigate the transition successfully.

Week 1: The Beginning of Change
In the initial week of transitioning to Dr. Sebi's alkaline diet, you'll be introducing your body to a new way of eating. Here's what you can expect:

Detoxification Signs

- **Fatigue:** As your body begins to detoxify, you may experience increased fatigue. This is common, and it's your body's way of conserving energy for the cleansing process.
- **Mild Headaches:** Some people report mild headaches as their bodies adjust to the absence of caffeine and processed foods.
- **Digestive Changes:** Your digestive system may need time to adapt to the increased intake of fiber from fruits and vegetables. This may result in alterations to bowel habits.

How to Navigate Week 1

- **Stay Hydrated:** Drinking plenty of water can help alleviate headaches and support the detox process.
- **Rest:** Embrace rest and prioritize sleep during this week. Your body needs extra energy for detoxification.

Week 2: Deepening Detox and Adjustment
During the second week, your body will further adjust to the alkaline diet, and the detoxification process will intensify:

Increased Detoxification: With a focus on deep cleansing, you might notice an increase in detox symptoms.

- **Skin Changes:** Some individuals experience breakouts or rashes as their skin eliminates toxins.
- **Improved Energy:** Although fatigue may continue, you may start to observe a gradual enhancement in your energy levels.

How to Navigate Week 2

- **Skin Care:** Gently cleanse and moisturize your skin to manage any breakouts or rashes.
- **Intermittent Fasting:** Consider incorporating intermittent fasting to support the detox process and give your digestive system a rest.
- **Embrace Herbal Supplements:** If you've opted for Dr. Sebi's herbal supplements, continue taking them as recommended. They can support various aspects of your health and detoxification journey.

Week 3: Nourishing Your Body
In Week 3, your focus will shift to nourishing your body with alkaline foods and balancing your nutrient intake:

Diverse Alkaline Foods: As you continue to expand your alkaline food choices, you'll discover a broader variety of fruits, nuts, vegetables, seeds, and whole grains.

- **Hydration:** You'll prioritize hydration with alkaline water and herbal teas, which are essential for supporting detoxification.
- **Emotional Well-Being:** This week emphasizes mental and emotional wellness as you become more attuned to your body's responses to the alkaline diet.

How to Navigate Week 3

- **Meal Planning:** Develop a meal planning routine to ensure you maintain a balanced and nutrient-rich diet.

- **Stress Management:** Continue practicing stress management techniques, like mindfulness and relaxation exercises.

Week 4: Establishing the Lifestyle
In the final week, you'll focus on solidifying the principles of Dr. Sebi's alkaline diet and making them part of your long-term lifestyle:

Integration and Consistency: The emphasis is on integrating the diet into your daily life and maintaining consistency.

- **Meal Planning:** You'll continue to prioritize meal planning, ensuring that you can sustain the detox lifestyle even during busy days.
- **Stress Management:** Managing stress through mindfulness and relaxation techniques remains crucial.

How to Navigate Week 4:

- **Support Network:** Connect with a support network of like-minded individuals following the alkaline diet. Sharing your experiences & challenges with others can be motivating.
- **Patience and Persistence:** Understand that challenges may still arise, but your commitment to the lifestyle you're establishing will help you overcome them.

Common Experiences During the Transition:
Throughout the entire 4-week transition process, you may encounter several common experiences:

1. **Cravings:** It's normal to experience cravings for familiar, non-alkaline foods, especially if your previous diet was high in sugar, salt, or processed components.

How to Navigate Cravings:

- As mentioned earlier, discover nutritious alternatives for your cravings. For instance, when you're yearning for something sweet, consider choosing fresh fruit. If you find yourself missing salty snacks, experiment with roasted nuts or seaweed snacks as satisfying options.
- Practice mindful eating. Taking time to savor your food could aid in decreasing cravings.

2. **Digestive Changes:** Shifting to an alkaline diet can lead to digestive changes. You may experience more frequent bowel movements, bloating, or other digestive discomforts.

How to Navigate Digestive Changes:

- Gradually increase your fiber intake to help your digestive system adapt to the change. Foods like chia seeds, flaxseeds, and leafy greens can be excellent sources of fiber.
- Ensure you're drinking plenty of water to stay hydrated, which is essential for healthy digestion.
3. **Emotional Changes:** Detoxification can lead to emotional changes, including mood swings and irritability.

How to Navigate Emotional Changes:

- Participate in mindfulness practices like meditation, yoga, or deep breathing exercises to effectively cope with stress and emotional fluctuations.
- Seek support from friends, family, or online communities to share your experiences and receive encouragement.
4. **Support Network:** Building a support network is crucial during the transition. Connecting with like-minded individuals can help you stay motivated and overcome challenges together.

How to Build a Support Network:

- Join online communities or local groups dedicated to the alkaline diet. Sharing your journey and seeking support can boost your commitment.
- Educate your friends and family about your dietary choices, so they can provide understanding and encouragement.

Remember, everyone's experience during the transition to Dr. Sebi's alkaline diet is unique. Listen to your body, stay patient with yourself, and seek professional guidance if needed. Over time, the positive changes in your health and well-being will likely outweigh any initial challenges you face. As you continue this journey, you'll likely find that the benefits of this lifestyle far outweigh the challenges, leading to a healthier and more vibrant you.

Common Mistakes and How to Avoid Them

Transitioning from a standard diet to Dr. Sebi's alkaline diet is a significant step toward improving your health and overall well-being. However, there are common mistakes that individuals often make during this transition. Understanding these mistakes and learning how to avoid them can help you navigate the journey more successfully.

Mistake 1: Insufficient Preparation and Education

- **Education:** Take the time to educate yourself about Dr. Sebi's alkaline diet. Understand the principles, the rationale behind it, and the specific foods that are encouraged and discouraged. Knowledge is your most potent tool.
- **Meal Planning:** Plan your meals in advance. This not only ensures that you have access to alkaline-friendly foods but also prevents you from being caught off guard and reaching for non-alkaline options.

Mistake 2: Sudden and Drastic Dietary Changes

- **Gradual Transition:** Instead of making abrupt and extreme dietary changes, consider a gradual transition. Begin by incorporating more alkaline foods into your current diet and progressively reducing acidic ones. This approach is more sustainable and eases the detox process on your body.
- **Consult a Healthcare Professional:** If you have underlying health conditions or dietary concerns, consult a registered dietitian or healthcare professional to ensure a safe and appropriate transition.

Mistake 3: Neglecting Proper Hydration

- **Prioritize Hydration:** Adequate hydration is crucial for the alkaline diet, as it helps support the detox process and maintain overall health. Consume alkaline water, herbal teas, and fresh fruit juices to ensure proper hydration.

- **Monitor Electrolytes:** Be aware of your electrolyte balance. The alkaline diet can affect electrolyte levels, so comprise foods high in potassium, like avocados and bananas, to help maintain balance.

Mistake 4: Focusing Solely on Food Choices

- **Incorporate Lifestyle Changes:** Dr. Sebi's alkaline diet is not just about food; it's a holistic lifestyle. Focus on other aspects of your lifestyle, like stress management, exercise, and getting adequate rest.

Mistake 5: Overlooking Nutritional Balance

- **Balanced Nutrition:** Pay attention to achieving a balanced intake of macronutrients (carbohydrates, protein, and healthy fats) from plant-based sources. This ensures you get a well-rounded set of nutrients.

- **Consult a Dietitian:** Should you have any concerns regarding meeting particular nutritional needs, it is advisable to reach out to a registered dietitian or nutritionist. They possess the knowledge and skills required to aid you in developing comprehensive meal plans and addressing any potential nutritional shortfalls or deficiencies, ensuring your diet remains wholesome and balanced.

Mistake 6: Not Incorporating Enough Variety

- **Diverse Diet:** The alkaline diet emphasizes a diverse and colorful diet. Incorporate a broad diversity of fruits, nuts, vegetables, and seeds to ensure you cover a broad spectrum of nutrients. Don't stick to a limited set of foods; explore new options regularly.

Mistake 7: Lack of Meal Planning

- **Meal Planning:** Plan your meals in advance to ensure you have access to alkaline-friendly options. This not only simplifies your diet but also prevents you from making impulsive, non-alkaline food choices.

Mistake 8: Skipping Herbal Supplements

- **Consider Supplements:** While the primary focus should be on food, Dr. Sebi's herbal supplements are designed to complement your diet and enhance detoxification. Depending on your needs and preferences, you may choose to include these supplements in your routine.

Mistake 9: Not Communicating Dietary Choices

- **Communication:** Let your friends and family know about your dietary choices and the reasons behind them. Educating them about your commitment can reduce social pressure and misunderstandings.
- **Prepare Your Own Dishes:** When you're participating in social gatherings or family events, volunteering to prepare a dish that adheres to your dietary preferences is a great strategy. This guarantees you'll have a meal that aligns with your dietary goals and helps make the event more enjoyable for you.

Mistake 10: Neglecting Stress Management

- **Stress Reduction Techniques:** Prioritize stress management techniques like meditation, yoga, deep breathing exercises, or any other practices that help you stay relaxed and emotionally balanced.

Mistake 11: Unrealistic Expectations

- **Realistic Goals:** Understand that transitioning to Dr. Sebi's alkaline diet is a process. Set realistic goals and expectations for your journey. You may encounter challenges, but with perseverance, you'll achieve long-term success.

Mistake 12: Lack of Patience

- **Be Patient:** The transition to an alkaline diet may involve adapting to changes in your body, including detoxification. Be patient with yourself, and remember that it's a journey with gradual improvements in your health and well-being.

Mistake 13: Neglecting Your Unique Needs

- **Listen to Your Body:** Pay close attention to how your body responds to the alkaline diet. Everyone is unique, and you may need to make adjustments to cater to your specific dietary requirements.

Mistake 14: Forgetting the Bigger Picture

- **Focus on the Long-Term:** Keep in mind the broader perspective of your health and well-being. Dr. Sebi's alkaline diet is not just about immediate results but about long-term benefits and a healthier lifestyle.

Avoiding these common mistakes and staying mindful of the key principles of Dr. Sebi's alkaline diet will significantly enhance your chances of a successful transition. Remember that it's a journey with the potential for profound health improvements, and as you continue to embrace this lifestyle, you'll likely find the benefits far outweigh any initial challenges.

Tips for a Smooth Transition

Transitioning from a standard diet to Dr. Sebi's alkaline diet can be a transformative and rewarding journey for your health and well-being. To ensure a smooth transition, it's essential to have a plan and a clear understanding of the diet's principles.

1. **Educate Yourself**

Before embarking on any dietary change, it's crucial to educate yourself about the principles and guidelines of Dr. Sebi's alkaline diet. Understanding the "what" and "why" behind this diet will empower you to make informed choices and ensure a smooth transition.

Key points to explore:

- **Alkaline vs. Acidic Foods:** Learn which foods are considered alkaline-forming and which are acidic. Focus on incorporating alkaline foods into your diet while reducing or eliminating acidic ones.

2. **Gradual Transition**

Rather than making a sudden and drastic change, consider a gradual transition. Start by integrating more alkaline foods into your current diet while reducing acidic and processed options over time. This approach lets your body to adjust gradually and minimizes potential detoxification symptoms.

3. **Meal Planning**

Meal planning is a cornerstone of success when transitioning to the alkaline diet. Planning your meals in advance ensures that you have access to alkaline-friendly options and reduces the temptation to opt for non-alkaline foods when you're in a rush or feeling hungry.

Tips for effective meal planning:

- Develop a weekly meal plan that encompasses a range of alkaline foods.
- Compile a shopping list according to your meal plan to guarantee you have the required components readily available.

- Consider batch cooking on weekends to have healthy, prepared meals throughout the week.

4. **Diverse and Colorful Diet**

The alkaline diet emphasizes the importance of consuming a broad diversity of fruits, vegetables, nuts, seeds, and whole grains. A diverse and colorful diet ensures you receive a broad spectrum of nutrients and phytonutrients.

Guidelines for a diverse diet:

- Incorporate different types of fruits and vegetables, aiming for a rainbow of colors on your plate.
- Explore new foods and components regularly to keep your meals exciting and nutrient-rich.

5. **Prioritize Hydration**

Adequate hydration is essential for the alkaline diet, as it supports the detoxification process and overall health. Consume alkaline water, herbal teas, and fresh fruit juices to ensure proper hydration.

Hydration tips:

- Consider acquiring a high-quality water filter to ensure that your drinking water is devoid of contaminants.
- Infuse your water with slices of alkaline-forming fruits like lemon, lime, or cucumber for added flavor.

6. **Mindful Eating**

Mindful eating entails focusing on your food, relishing each bite, and staying fully engaged during your meals. This practice can help you make conscious, health-focused food choices and prevent overeating.

- How to incorporate mindful eating:
- Turn off distractions like the TV or phone while eating.
- Chew your food thoroughly and take your time to relish the flavors and textures of your meal.

7. **Herbal Supplements**

Dr. Sebi's herbal supplements are designed to complement the alkaline diet and enhance the detoxification process. Depending on your specific health goals and preferences, you may choose to include these supplements in your routine.

Steps for using herbal supplements:

- Seek guidance from a healthcare professional or herbalist to ascertain which supplements are appropriate for your specific requirements.
- Adhere to the suggested dosages and instructions for each supplement.

8. **Support Network**

Building a support network can be tremendously advantageous as you transition to the alkaline diet. Connect with individuals who share similar dietary goals. Sharing your experiences & challenges with others can offer encouragement and motivation.

Ways to build a support network:

- Join online communities or local groups dedicated to the alkaline diet.
- Share your journey with friends and family, and encourage them to participate in or support your dietary choices.

9. **Be Patient with Yourself**

Remember that transitioning to Dr. Sebi's alkaline diet is a journey, not a destination. Be patient with yourself and understand that it's natural to encounter challenges along the way. Embrace the learning process and focus on the long-term benefits of this lifestyle.

Tips for practicing patience:

- Set realistic short-term and long-term goals to help you stay motivated.
- Celebrate your achievements, no matter how small they may seem.

10. Stress Management

Stress management is an integral part of the alkaline diet. Chronic stress can have adverse impacts on your health, making it crucial to prioritize relaxation and stress-reduction strategies.

Effective stress management strategies:

- Incorporate regular meditation or mindfulness practices into your daily routine.
- Engage in physical activities like yoga, deep breathing exercises, or nature walks to reduce stress.

11. Seek Professional Guidance

If you're dealing with specific health concerns, dietary restrictions, or underlying medical conditions, it's a wise choice to consult with a registered dietitian, nutritionist, or healthcare professional who specializes in plant-based diets. Their specialized knowledge can be a valuable resource, allowing them to provide personalized guidance to suit your individual needs and helping you navigate your dietary choices effectively.

Guidelines for seeking professional guidance:

- Talk about your health objectives and concerns with your healthcare provider.
- Be open to recommendations and advice tailored to your unique needs.

12. **Stay Committed to Your Goals**

The success of your transition to the alkaline diet depends on your commitment. Clearly define your reasons for adopting this diet and remind yourself of your goals regularly. Staying committed will help you overcome challenges and reap the long-term benefits of this lifestyle.

Strategies for maintaining commitment:

- Keep a journal to track your progress & reflect on how the diet is benefiting your health and well-being.
- Connect with your support network to stay motivated and accountable.

Chapter 7:

Lifelong Alkaline Affair

Congratulations on successfully completing the 28-Day Detox Plan! You've come a long way in your journey towards embracing Dr. Sebi's Alkaline and Anti-Inflammatory Diet. You've already experienced the benefits of reducing acidity and inflammation in your body, and now it's time to delve deeper into this lifelong alkaline affair.

In this chapter, we'll explore what lies beyond the initial detox and dive into holistic approaches for maintaining a balanced alkaline lifestyle. This is not just a diet; it's a lifelong commitment to your health and well-being. We'll guide you through incorporating physical exercise and making healthy lifestyle choices to ensure you stay on the path to optimal health.

Beyond the 28-Day Plan

Dr. Sebi's 28-Day Detox Plan is a fantastic starting point for transforming your health and reducing inflammation in your body. It has provided you with the foundations of an alkaline lifestyle and allowed you to experience the benefits firsthand. However, it's essential to understand that the 28-day plan is just the beginning of your journey. To truly embrace the alkaline lifestyle, you need to commit to it for the long term.

1. **Gradual Transition**

After completing the detox, it's crucial to transition into a sustainable, long-term alkaline diet gradually. This transition phase helps your body adjust to this new way of eating. Start by reintroducing foods that are still within the alkaline spectrum but were restricted during the detox. This will allow you to have a more diverse and balanced diet while still maintaining the principles of Dr. Sebi's diet.

The 28-Day Detox Plan was a period of strict adherence to alkaline foods to kickstart the process of reducing acidity and inflammation in your body. However, it's not a sustainable long-term diet. The transition phase after the detox is an essential step to gradually reintroduce a broader range of alkaline foods into your diet.

The key to a successful transition is to do it gradually. Reintroduce one type of food at a time and monitor how your body responds. For example, you might start with introducing specific fruits or vegetables that were not part of the detox plan. Gradually include them to your meals and observe how your body reacts. This approach allows you to identify any foods that may not agree with your system and make adjustments accordingly.

Remember that the goal is to create a balanced, sustainable diet that is still primarily alkaline but allows for more variety in your daily meals. By doing this gradually, you'll find a way of eating that works for you in the long term and is enjoyable to maintain.

2. **Continual Learning**

One of the keys to a lifelong alkaline affair is knowledge. Keep educating yourself about alkaline foods, their benefits, and how to incorporate them into your daily life. Continue reading and researching to stay informed and motivated. The more you know, the better equipped you'll be to make informed dietary choices.

Learning about the science behind the alkaline diet, the health benefits it offers, and the specific properties of various alkaline foods will empower you to make more informed choices. While you don't need to become a nutrition expert, having a solid understanding of the principles behind the diet can help you make better decisions.

Stay updated on the latest research related to alkaline diets and health. Knowledge is your greatest tool in maintaining a lifelong alkaline lifestyle. Consider reading books, following reputable websites, and staying connected with communities that share your commitment to this way of life.

3. **Accountability and Support**

Joining support groups or seeking the guidance of a certified nutritionist can be incredibly beneficial. These tools foster a feeling of belonging and responsibility, helping to keep you motivated and on course. Being in the company of individuals who share your goals can enhance the experience and make it more enduring.

Having someone to hold you accountable and providing you with support may result in an enormous impact in your ability to sustain an alkaline lifestyle. Whether you find an online community, attend local support groups, or work with a certified nutritionist, having a network of individuals who understand your journey can be immensely motivating.

Support groups offer a forum for exchanging experiences, obstacles, and achievements. They can offer practical tips, answer questions, and provide a sense of belonging. Additionally, you can learn from others who have been on this path for a longer time, benefiting from their knowledge and insights.

Nutritionists with expertise in the alkaline diet can offer personalized guidance. They can help you create meal plans, identify foods that work best for your body, and address any specific health concerns or dietary restrictions you may have. Collaborating with a nutritionist can represent a worthwhile commitment to your overall well-being in the long run.

Holistic Approaches for a Balanced Life

A holistic approach to maintaining an alkaline lifestyle involves more than just dietary choices. It's about embracing a comprehensive, well-rounded way of living that promotes overall health and well-being. Let's explore some key aspects of this holistic approach.

1. **Regular Exercise**

Physical activity is a crucial component of an alkaline lifestyle. Physical activity aids not just in weight management but also in facilitating your body's natural detoxification processes. It boosts your metabolism and strengthens your immune system, reducing the risk of chronic diseases.

Integrate consistent exercise into your daily schedule, striving for a minimum of 150 mins of moderate-intensity aerobic activity each week. Activities like brisk walking, cycling, and swimming are excellent choices. Additionally, consider adding strength training exercises to build lean muscle and further boost your metabolism.

Physical activity plays a vital role in sustaining an equilibrium within an alkaline lifestyle. It complements a nutritious diet to foster overall health. Regular exercise provides a plethora of advantages, including weight control, better cardiovascular fitness, and an uplifted mood.

Aim to create a workout routine that you relish and can stick to. This might involve a mix of aerobic exercises like walking, jogging, or cycling and strength training exercises that focus on building and toning your muscles. If you're just beginning to incorporate exercise into your routine, begin at a comfortable pace and slowly ramp up the intensity as your fitness level progresses.

Exercise not only supports your overall health but also contributes to maintaining a balanced pH in your body. When you engage in physical activity, your muscles produce acids as a byproduct of energy metabolism. These acids can contribute to an acidic environment in your body. However, regular exercise also enhances your body's ability to take out these acids, ultimately helping you maintain a more alkaline state.

2. **Stress Management**

Stress can trigger inflammation in the body, hindering progress on your alkaline journey. Practicing stress management techniques like meditation, deep breathing exercises, and mindfulness could aid in decreasing the negative impact of stress on your health. Make time for relaxation and self-care to maintain emotional well-being.

Stress management is a vital aspect of maintaining an alkaline lifestyle. Persistent stress can negatively affect your health, resulting in heightened inflammation and acidity within the body. Therefore, incorporating stress-reduction techniques is essential for promoting overall well-being.

Various stress management techniques can help you maintain emotional balance and reduce the physiological effects of stress on your body. Some effective methods include:

- **Meditation:** To achieve mental clarity and relaxation, the practice of meditation includes concentrating one's attention on a single object, train of thought, or activity in particular. Consistent meditation practice has demonstrated its ability to diminish stress, enhance emotional well-being, and foster a profound sense of tranquility.

- **Deep Breathing Exercises:** Techniques like diaphragmatic breathing can effectively soothe your nervous system, reduce stress hormone levels, and alleviate tension. Devoting a few mins each day to practicing deep breathing exercises can significantly reduce your stress levels.
- **Mindfulness:** Mindfulness involves keenly observing the present moment without passing judgment. This method can elevate your mindfulness regarding your thoughts and emotions, empowering you to react to stressors in a more positive way.
- **Yoga:** Relaxation and stress reduction are two of the primary goals of yoga, which is achieved through a combination of physical postures, breathing exercises, and meditation. Regular yoga practice can improve flexibility, reduce tension, and enhance emotional well-being.

Integrating these stress-reduction practices into your daily regimen can assist you in preserving emotional equilibrium and diminishing the physical repercussions of stress on your body. Whether it's through a formal meditation practice or simple deep breathing exercises, finding ways to manage stress is crucial for your overall well-being.

3. **Ample Hydration**

Staying hydrated is a fundamental part of the alkaline lifestyle. Water is essential for maintaining the body's pH balance and supporting various bodily functions. Aim to drink at least 8 glasses of water a day and consider incorporating alkaline water, which can have a more favorable pH level.

Hydration is a key component of maintaining a balanced alkaline lifestyle. Water plays a critical role in regulating your body's pH, and staying well-hydrated is essential for supporting various physiological processes.

Strive to consume a minimum of 8 glasses of water daily. Nevertheless, it's essential to recognize that individual hydration requirements may differ depending on factors like climate, physical activity, and overall well-being. It's essential to listen to your body and consume water as needed. Pay attention to signs of dehydration, like dark urine, dry mouth, or feelings of thirst.

In addition to regular water, you may also consider incorporating alkaline water into your daily routine. Alkaline water has a higher pH level than regular tap water, making it less acidic. Some proponents of the alkaline diet believe that consuming alkaline water can help balance the body's pH, although scientific evidence on this is still inconclusive. If you choose to explore alkaline water, consult with your healthcare provider and ensure that it aligns with your overall dietary plan.

4. Quality Sleep

Quality sleep is often overlooked but is crucial for maintaining an alkaline lifestyle. During sleep, your body repairs and rejuvenates itself. Aim for 7-9 hrs of uninterrupted, restful sleep each night. Create a sleep-conducive environment and establish a regular sleep schedule to promote better overall health.

Quality sleep is a cornerstone of maintaining an alkaline lifestyle. While diet and exercise are essential, the role of sleep in promoting overall well-being cannot be overstated. When you sleep, your body undergoes various restorative processes that support your health.

Target a sleep duration of 7-9 hrs per night. The specific amount of sleep needed can vary depending on individual factors, but this range is generally recommended for adults. Consistently getting enough sleep helps regulate hormones, repair tissues, and enhance cognitive function.

To promote quality sleep, consider the following tips:

- **Establish a consistent sleep schedule:** Make an effort to retire to bed and rise at the same times every day, even during weekends. Consistency aids in regulating your body's internal clock.
- **Create a conducive sleep environment:** Ensure that your bedroom is optimized for rest. Ensure that your room remains at a cool temperature, shrouded in darkness, and free of noise disturbances. Invest in a cozy mattress and pillows that accommodate your preferred sleeping position.
- **Reduce screen time:** Avoid screens for a minimum of one hour before bedtime, as the blue light emitted by electronic devices can disturb your sleep.
- **Employ relaxation techniques:** Partake in calming activities before bedtime to help you unwind. These activities may include reading, gentle stretches, or deep breathing exercises.
- **Watch your diet:** Be mindful of when and what you eat before bedtime. Heavy or spicy meals can disrupt sleep, so aim to finish eating at least a few hrs before bedtime.

By prioritizing sleep and creating a healthy sleep routine, you'll support your body's ability to maintain an alkaline state and overall well-being.

5. Mindful Living

Engaging in mindfulness entails immersing yourself completely in the current moment and deliberately making thoughtful decisions. Be mindful of what you eat, how you move, and how you live. This awareness can help you make better decisions in alignment with your alkaline lifestyle.

Mindful living is a foundational aspect of maintaining an alkaline lifestyle. Being fully present in the moment and making conscious choices in all aspects of your life can help you align your actions with your health goals.

Here are some ways to incorporate mindful living into your daily routine:

- **Mindful Eating:** Pay close attention to the foods you consume. Take your time to chew your food slowly and relish each mouthful. This practice can help you recognize when you're full, preventing overeating.
- **Mindful Exercise:** When you engage in physical activity, be present in the moment. Focus on the sensations in your body, your breath, and the movements you're making. This can enhance your exercise experience and make it more enjoyable.
- **Mindful Choices:** Consider how your daily choices align with your health goals. Are your actions supporting your commitment to an alkaline lifestyle? By regularly assessing your choices, you can make adjustments as needed.
- **Mindful Stress Management:** When practicing stress-reduction techniques, like meditation or deep breathing exercises, fully engage in the process. Allow yourself to let go of distractions and immerse yourself in the practice.

By incorporating mindfulness into your daily life, you'll become more attuned to your body's needs and better equipped to make choices that support your alkaline lifestyle.

By embracing the principles outlined in this chapter, you're embarking on a lifelong alkaline affair. It's not just about a diet; it's a comprehensive way of living that prioritizes your health and well-being. The benefits you've experienced during the 28-Day Detox Plan are just the beginning of what's possible.

Maintaining a balanced alkaline lifestyle is an ongoing journey, and it's one that can be incredibly rewarding. It's a commitment to a healthier, happier you. With dedication and mindful choices, you can relish the rewards of optimal health for years to come.

Remember that every individual's journey is unique, and what works best for one person may not work for another. Your path to a lifelong alkaline affair is a personal one. It's about discovering what aligns with your values, preferences, and needs while staying true to the principles of Dr. Sebi's Alkaline and Anti-Inflammatory Diet.

As you continue this journey, keep learning, adapting, and exploring new ways to maintain your alkaline lifestyle. You have the power to make choices that will positively impact your health, reduce inflammation in your body, and support a long and fulfilling life.

Conclusion: The Horizon of Holistic Harmony

In conclusion, our voyage through the realm of holistic well-being has been a profound and enlightening exploration of the path to a life filled with vibrancy, energy, and the soothing whispers of nature. This journey is not one with a final destination; rather, it is a continuous expedition towards health, vitality, and the profound sense of well-being that we all seek.

Throughout this guide, we have embarked on a comprehensive exploration of holistic living. We have ventured into the nurturing of physical, mental, emotional, and spiritual well-being, and have delved deep into the world of holistic healing practices. The recurring theme that has emerged is the profound interconnectedness of these various facets of our existence. To achieve a life of balance and harmony, it is essential to tend to each of these dimensions.

As we take a moment to reflect on this expedition, it's crucial to understand that the pursuit of holistic well-being is not about reaching a state of perfection. It is about making progress, no matter how small or large, and embracing your unique journey. Each step forward is a step toward a healthier, more vibrant life, and it is guided by your values, needs, and aspirations.

A Lifelong Journey to Health

The journey to holistic harmony is anything but linear. It is an ongoing process of self-discovery, personal growth, and continuous self-improvement. Each challenge faced is an opportunity for growth, and your commitment to holistic well-being will be your compass on this remarkable voyage. Whether life presents obstacles or opportunities, your dedication to holistic well-being will lead you to a life that radiates with vibrancy and vitality, much like the ever-changing beauty of the natural world.

The voyage towards health, vitality, and a profound sense of well-being is a lifelong commitment, but it is a commitment that is profoundly rewarding. As you gaze into the horizon of your life, understand that you possess the tools and knowledge needed to navigate the complex seas of well-being with grace and resilience. Embracing the interconnectedness of your existence and nurturing each aspect of your being, including the physical, mental, emotional, and spiritual dimensions, will bring you closer to the harmonious life you aspire to lead.

May your journey be filled with joy, vitality, and an ever-deepening connection to the abundant beauty that surrounds you. The horizon of holistic harmony stretches infinitely, offering limitless opportunities for exploration, discovery, and savoring. As you continue your journey, let your life present as a testament to the profound power of holistic living and its transformative influence on your well-being and the world around you.

In this pursuit of holistic well-being, you have become the captain of your own ship, steering through the unpredictable waters of life. You have acquired the wisdom to discern which winds to harness and which storms to weather. With each choice made in favor of your holistic well-being, you move closer to the life of balance, harmony, and vitality you desire. Your journey, like the tides and seasons, will ebb and flow, but your commitment to holistic well-being will remain a constant guiding star.

In closing, remember that the voyage to holistic harmony is not one with an endpoint. It is a journey that extends beyond the horizon, where new vistas of well-being and self-discovery await. As you continue on your path, may you find not only the harmony you seek within yourself but also the capacity to inspire and uplift those around you, demonstrating the extraordinary potential of holistic living. Your life is a testament to the holistic harmony you pursue, and its ripple effect will touch the lives of others, making the world a better place, one harmonious soul at a time.

Index

Red Pepper Rejuvenation Juice; 88

Spinach and Pineapple Green Smoothie; 78

Spinach Sunshine Elixir; 97

Strawberry Fields Forever Juice; 93

Sweet Potato Spice Smoothie; 80

Turmeric Pineapple Passion; 98

Watermelon Wonder Juice; 79

Scan the QR code to access the link to download your bonus!

Made in the USA
Coppell, TX
10 May 2024

32216525R00075